Free Video  **Free Video**

Essential Test Tips Video from Trivium Test Prep

Dear Customer,

Thank you for purchasing from Trivium Test Prep! We're honored to help you prepare for your CCM exam.

To show our appreciation, we're offering a **FREE CCM *Essential Test Tips* Video by Trivium Test Prep.*** Our video includes 35 test preparation strategies that will make you successful on the CCM. All we ask is that you email us your feedback and describe your experience with our product. Amazing, awful, or just so-so: we want to hear what you have to say!

To receive your **FREE CCM *Essential Test Tips* Video**, please email us at 5star@ triviumtestprep.com. Include "Free 5 Star" in the subject line and the following information in your email:

1. The title of the product you purchased.
2. Your rating from 1 – 5 (with 5 being the best).
3. Your feedback about the product, including how our materials helped you meet your goals and ways in which we can improve our products.
4. Your full name and shipping address so we can send your **FREE CCM *Essential Test Tips* Video.**

If you have any questions or concerns please feel free to contact us directly at 5star@ triviumtestprep.com.

Thank you!

– Trivium Test Prep Team

*To get access to the free video please email us at 5star@triviumtestprep.com, and please follow the instructions above.

CCM CERTIFICATION STUDY GUIDE 2019–2020

Certified Case Manager Test Preparation and Practice Questions for the CCM Certification Exam

TABLE OF CONTENTS

ONLINE RESOURCES

To help you fully prepare for your Certified Case Management (CCM) exam, Ascencia includes online resources with the purchase of this study guide.

Practice Test

In addition to the practice test included in this book, we also offer an online exam. Since many exams today are computer based, getting to practice your test-taking skills on the computer is a great way to prepare.

Flash Cards

A convenient supplement to this study guide, Ascencia's flash cards enable you to review important terms easily on your computer or smartphone.

Cheat Sheets

Review the core skills you need to master the exam with easy-to-read Cheat Sheets.

From Stress to Success

Watch "From Stress to Success," a brief but insightful YouTube video that offers the tips, tricks, and secrets experts use to score higher on the exam.

Reviews

Leave a review, send us helpful feedback, or sign up for Ascencia promotions—including free books!

Access these materials at: **www.ascenciatestprep.com/ccm-online-resources**

INTRODUCTION

Congratulations on choosing to take the Certified Case Manager (CCM) Exam! Passing the CCM is an important step forward in your health care career.

In the following pages, you will find information about the CCM, what to expect on test day, how to use this book, and the content covered on the exam.

The CCMC Certification Process

The **Certified Case Manager (CCM) Exam** is developed by the **Commission for Case Manager Certification (CCMC)** as part of its certification program for case managers. The CCM measures the skills necessary to excel as a case manager in a variety of health care settings. To qualify for the exam, you must have a current licensure in any health or human services discipline permitting independent assessment of a client in the United States or its territories. Instead of licensure, you may qualify if you have a bachelor's or advanced degree in certain health or human services disciplines.

You must also have employment experience: either twelve months of case management experience under the supervision of a board-certified case manager, twelve months of experience supervising case managers, or twenty-four months of full-time case management experience. All experience must be obtained in the United States.

Once you have met the qualifications and passed the exam, you will have your CCM certification, and you may use the credentials as long as your certification is valid. You will need to recertify every five years. You can earn your recertification by taking continuing education courses or by retaking the exam. If you are taking the exam for recertification, you must take the exam before the "valid through" date on your certificate.

CCM Questions and Timing

The CCM consists of **180 questions**. Only 150 of these questions are scored; thirty are unscored, or *pretest* questions. These questions are included by the CCMC to test their suitability for inclusion in future tests. You'll have no way of knowing which questions are unscored, so treat every question like it counts.

The questions on the CCM are multiple-choice with four answer choices. The CCM has **no-guess penalty**. That is, if you answer a question incorrectly, no points are deducted from your score; you simply do not get credit for that question. Therefore, you should always guess if you do not know the answer to a question.

You will have **three hours** to complete the test. Before the timed portion of the exam begins, you will take a brief tutorial. There are no scheduled breaks during the exam.

CCM Content Areas

The CCMC conducts ongoing research to determine the content of the CCM exam. The CCM exam is based on five major domains of essential knowledge for case managers, corresponding to the **Five Core Components of Case Management**. Case managers are typically responsible for assessment, planning, implementation, coordination, monitoring, and evaluation, using core knowledge areas from the five core components. The table below gives the five major domains of essential knowledge and a breakdown of the questions on the exam.

Quick Summary of CCM Test Sections		
Section	**Percentage of the Exam**	**Approx. No. of Questions**
Care Delivery and Reimbursement Methods	31%	47
Psychosocial Concepts and Support Systems	27%	40
Quality and Outcomes Evaluation and Measurements	18%	27
Rehabilitation Concepts and Strategies	9%	13
Ethical, Legal, and Practice Standards	15%	23
Total		**150 questions**

Care Delivery and Reimbursement Methods questions make up the bulk of the exam, addressing the goals and objectives of case management practice and case management processes and tools. Questions address the roles and functions of case managers and other providers in various settings, the continuum of care/continuum of health and human services, the interdisciplinary care team (ICT), and client adherence to care regimen. Prepare for questions about managing acute and chronic illness and disability and managing clients with multiple chronic illnesses, including medication therapy management and reconciliation. Be aware of factors used to identify a client's acuity or severity levels; physical functioning and behavioral health assessment may also be addressed. Expect questions on managed care concepts; health care delivery systems and providers; levels of care and care settings; and transitions of care. Questions will specifically address alternative care facilities like assisted living, group homes, residential treatment facilities; behavioral health and community vendors; different models of care like patient-centered medical homes (PCMHs), accountable care organizations, health homes, special needs plans (SNPs), and the chronic care model; and hospice, palliative, and end-of-life care.

These questions also address reimbursement and payment methodologies (e.g., bundled, case rate, prospective payment systems, and value-based purchasing). Expect to see questions about benefit programs. Questions on private benefits programs cover issues like employer-sponsored health coverage, individual-purchased insurance, home care benefits, COBRA, pharmacy benefits management, and indemnity. Public programs like SSI, SSDI, Medicare, and Medicaid are also addressed. Be prepared for questions about military benefit programs as well (TRICARE, VA, etc.). General insurance principles like health, disability, workers compensation, and long-term care are addressed, as are cost containment principles and other financial resources (waiver programs, special needs trusts, and viatical settlements). Expect questions on negotiation techniques and utilization management principles and guidelines. You should also prepare for questions on coding methodologies, including diagnosis-related group (DRG), *The Diagnostic and Statistical Manual of Mental Disorders (DSM)*, the International Classification of Diseases (ICD), and Current Procedural Terminology (CPT).

Psychosocial Concepts and Support Systems questions address the psychosocial aspects of chronic illness and disability. These questions are the second-largest portion of the exam. They include psychological and neuropsychological assessment; behavioral health concepts like dual diagnoses; substance use, abuse, and addiction; behavioral change theories; and abuse and neglect. Community resources like elder care services, fraternal or religious organizations, government programs, meal delivery services, and pharmacy assistance programs; other resources for the uninsured or underinsured; and other support programs like support groups, pastoral counseling, and bereavement counseling are also covered. Prepare for questions on end-of-life issues, spirituality (as related to health behavior), and cultural and religious factors that may affect a client's health status. Interpersonal communication, conflict resolution and crisis intervention strategies, and family dynamics are also addressed. Questions may focus on client engagement, empowerment, and self-care management; health coaching; interview techniques; and wellness strategies.

Quality and Outcomes Evaluation and Measurements questions address issues like data interpretation and reporting, cost-benefit analysis, caseload calculation, program evaluation and methodology, quality and performance improvement, and accreditation standards and requirements. Health care analytics, such as health risk assessment, predictive modeling, and Adjusted Clinical Group (ACG) may be covered. Be prepared for questions about *sources* of quality indicators like the Centers for Medicare and Medicaid Services (CMS), the Utilization Review Accreditation Commission (URAC), the National Committee for Quality Assurance (NCQA), the National Quality Forum (NQF), and the Agency for Healthcare Research and Quality (AHRQ). Types of quality indicators (clinical, financial, productivity, utilization, quality, client experience) may also be addressed.

Rehabilitation Concepts and Strategies questions focus on the vocational aspects of chronic illness and disability, including vocational and rehabilitation service delivery systems. Rehabilitation (post-injury, including work injury, post-hospitalization, or acute health condition) and functional capacity evaluations are covered. Expect some questions on assistive devices like prosthetics, text telephone device, teletypewriter (TTY), telecommunications device for the Deaf (TDD), and orientation and mobility services.

Ethical, Legal, and Practice Standards questions ask about ethics related to care delivery (e.g., advocacy, experimental treatments and protocols, end of life, refusal of treatment/services) and professional practice (e.g., code of conduct, veracity). These questions also address legal and regulatory requirements, and health care and disability-related legislation like the Americans with Disabilities Act (ADA), OSHA regulations, the Health Insurance Portability and Accountability Act (HIPAA), and the Affordable Care Act (ACA). Other topics might include case recording and documentation; privacy and confidentiality; meaningful use; risk management; critical pathways; standards of care, practice guidelines, and treatment guidelines; self-care and well-being as a professional; and standards of practice.

For the most current information on the exam, check the CCMC at https://ccmcertification.org/.

Exam Administration

To register for the exam, you must first apply through the CCMC (https://ccmcertification.org/get-certified/certification). After your application is accepted, you will receive an exam eligibility email with your testing number and instructions on how to register for the exam. The exam is offered three times a year by Prometric. The email will contain instructions on how to schedule your exam appointment with Prometric.

The CCM is administered at Prometric testing centers around the nation. Plan to arrive at least **thirty minutes before the exam** to complete biometric screening. Bring at least one form of **government-issued photo ID** and be prepared to be photographed and have your fingertips scanned. You will also be scanned with a metal detector wand before entering the test room. Your primary ID must be government issued, include a recent photograph and signature, and match the name under which you registered to take the test. If you do not have proper ID, you will not be allowed to take the test.

You will not be allowed to bring any personal items into the testing room, such as calculators or phones. You may not bring pens, pencils, or scratch paper. Other prohibited items include hats, scarves, and coats. You may wear religious garments, however. Prometric provides lockers for valuables. You can keep your ID and locker key with you.

Exam Results

Once you have completed your test, the computer you are working on will display your pass/fail score. You may print a hard copy of your score to take with you. You will receive your official results electronically four weeks after the end of the testing window. Remember, you may not use your CCM credentials until you have received your official results, even if you pass the test.

The CCM is a pass/fail test. Of the 180 questions on the test, 150 are scored. Your raw score is how many of the 150 scored questions you answer correctly. That score is then scaled based on the level of difficulty of the questions you answered correctly. The minimum passing scaled score is 500. You will only receive a score report if you do NOT pass the exam. The report will include the candidate's score.

If you pass the test, you will receive a certificate in the mail about four weeks after the end of the testing window. You will not receive a score report if you pass.

The number of correct answers needed to pass the exam will vary slightly depending on the questions included in your version of the test (i.e., if you took a version of the test with harder questions, the passing score will be lower). For security reasons, different versions of the test are administered every testing window. For most test takers, **a passing score will be 105 questions answered correctly.** However, this can range from 105 to 110 questions.

Using This Book

This book is divided into two sections. In the content area review, you will find the pathophysiology, risk factors, signs and symptoms, diagnostic findings, and treatment protocols for the conditions included in the CCM framework. Throughout the chapter you'll also see Quick Review Questions that will help reinforce important concepts and skills.

The book also includes two full-length practice tests (one in the book and one online) with answer rationales. You can use these tests to gauge your readiness for the test and determine which content areas you may need to review more thoroughly.

Ascencia Test Prep

With health care fields such as nursing, pharmacy, emergency care, and physical therapy becoming the fastest-growing industries in the United States, individuals looking to enter the health care industry or rise in their field need high-quality, reliable resources. Ascencia Test Prep's study guides and test preparation materials are developed by credentialed industry professionals with years of experience in their respective fields. Ascencia recognizes that health care professionals nurture bodies and spirits, and save lives. Ascencia Test Prep's mission is to help health care workers grow.

ONE: CASE MANAGEMENT CONCEPTS

The Goals and Objectives of Case Management

A board-certified case manager (CCM) is a proud professional who has passed an exam to become nationally certified. All case managers have the common goal of serving as a client advocate. This role requires the CCM to ensure that clients receive the proper care and remain as safe and healthy as possible. The CCM will establish a care plan by assessing the needs of their client. Based on those needs, the CCM can perform a wide range of job duties, including educating clients and their families, attending physician appointments, obtaining medical equipment for rehabilitation, and researching medication assistance funding.

Typically, case managers are also nurses or social workers and can work in a variety of health care settings. These settings include hospitals, doctors' offices, and behavior health facilities. The CCM may work in the workers' compensation field or serve children or adults with disabilities.

Case management has four main goals:

+ improve quality of care
+ reduce health care costs
+ coordinate care
+ encourage client engagement and self-advocacy

Improvement of quality of care is an important task of the CCM. The CCM serves as another set of eyes for their client. Medical care can be overwhelming to a patient, who may leave the hospital without understanding what to do upon returning home. The CCM will assess the hospital discharge summary and educate the client on follow-up medical appointments or medications. Quality of care is achieved when the CCM assists their client with information that may be lacking or misunderstood.

Health care costs may be reduced by interventions to help the client avoid hospitalization. The CCM may observe that a client is not complying with their prescribed insulin usage, for example. The client simply may not know how to inject the insulin and therefore will return to the hospital with elevated blood sugar. A patient may need education on the importance and correct execution of behavior medications. Lack of education may lead to the patient having to enter a behavioral facility.

With many medical professionals often involved with caring for the same patient, care is overlooked or misunderstood at times. The CCM may assist a client by communicating with all medical professionals involved to ensure that everyone is "on the same page" by coordinating care. Also, many clients may need services or medical equipment and might not know how to meet these needs. For example, the CCM can help a mother obtain a wheelchair for her child at the best cost available through research and communication.

Encouragement is needed at times to achieve goals on the care plan created by the CCM. The client may wish to quit smoking, for example, but does not think it is possible. Researching community smoking cessation programs and being an extra resource for support may help a client to become engaged. Working on short- and long-term goals may be useful. Return demonstrations on medical equipment usage will ensure the client is using the equipment correctly. A CCM who engages in these actions and observes medication administration, will encourage client engagement and self-advocacy.

PRACTICE QUESTION

1.   A patient underwent cardiac surgery and is given instructions to rest from their physician. Which of the following actions would NOT promote the goals of case management?

     A) completing a medical reconciliation against the discharge papers
     B) finding transportation for the patient for medical appointments
     C) allowing the patient to rest while the CCM meets with providers
     D) researching lower-cost medications

The Case Management Process

The case management process includes a number of steps. First, it is necessary to determine eligibility of the case management services. The disease complexity of the client will be considered along with the frequency and setting of the CCM's visits. After a client is determined to be eligible for case management, the CCM will complete a comprehensive assessment to determine a plan of action to achieve the client's health care goals. Implementing the plan and following up to ensure client goals have been met will reduce health care costs to the client and society as a whole.

SCREENING

Due to the high cost of health care and increasing demand for it, not everyone will qualify for case management services. This specialty service is determined by a **screening** process, whereby insurance eligibility and client health status are reviewed. Items reviewed for eligibility include medical claims and the client's health and disability history, including current health condition and frequency of receiving medical treatment.

A **high utilizer** is a person who frequents the hospital or emergency department often and is likely to be eligible for case management services. This type of client may have multiple diseases and may lack the education necessary to avoid hospital admissions. Injured workers, disabled persons, and the chronic disease population are among those who may be eligible for case management services.

Client information can be entered into a system and screened by using a special program. The screening questions, sometimes called **Brief Intake**, will note red flags that increase eligibility for case management services. These red flags may include frequent emergency room visits (for issues such as hyperglycemia, shortness of breath, or fluid retention) or frequent hospitalizations (for issues such as repeated falls).

Determination of eligibility is made by insurance companies, human services departments, and government agencies such as Medicaid. After the client is determined eligible, the case manager will be notified by the company and provided client demographics.

STRATIFYING RISK

Stratifying risk determines the likelihood that an individual may incur higher medical claims. During this process, an individual is placed in a group based on the specific health-related screening answers they provide. These groups may be defined as high, moderate, or low. For example, a young female who exercises often and does not smoke may be placed into a low-risk group. In contrast, a sixty-three-year-old male who is diagnosed as diabetic with two hospital admissions within six months may be placed into a high-risk group.

The goal of stratifying risk is to identify a situation or risk before it becomes a problem, and direct resources toward it. This predictive data enables an intervention to be developed that may prevent future problems that would elevate medical costs. Clients in a low-risk group may simply need to see their primary doctor as advised and maintain wellness exams. Moderate- to high-risk groups will need more intensive interventions to maximize their well-being and minimize health care costs. The case manager may need to make home visits or telephone calls. For these clients, medication reconciliation and follow-up doctor appointments will be a priority.

ASSESSING

A CCM cannot advocate for their client without first **assessing** the needs of the client by using a health assessment. The answers to the assessment questions will provide the CCM with a clearer picture of the plan that needs to be formulated to assist the client in achieving their goals. The CCM will be assessing demographics, financial status, social needs, depression risks, caregivers used, and medical information. The client will provide all medical information as well as medications prescribed. Any legal documents related to care will also be discussed. The CCM will also want to know about wellness exams and financial concerns. This provides a complete picture of health maintenance knowledge and education needed. Many assessment questions will be directed toward how much personal grooming and self-care a patient can do alone.

> 🔍 During assessment, the case manager should be nonjudgmental. Remember, your purpose as a client's assigned CCM is to improve their health. If the client feels judged, they may feel ashamed and not answer the questions as honestly as possible.

Another important component of the assessment survey will be the family dynamics. Is there a family member who drives the client to doctors' appointments, or does the client drive? Is there a family member who the client would prefer the CCM meet with? The family member is often quite valuable in assessing client needs.

After completing an assessment, the CCM will be able to compile a list of the client's needs. The CCM can then dive into helping the client achieve their health care goals.

PLANNING

Planning a strategy is vital for achieving the client's health-related goals. The CCM will use the list of needs discovered from the client assessment to create a care plan. A good **care plan** will include:

+ the problem noted
+ the goal to be achieved
+ interventions the CCM will use
+ evaluation of the intervention

An example of a care plan for a diabetic client may deal with diabetic foot monitoring and treatment. The goal will be a measurable one with a realistic time frame, such as "The patient will demonstrate the importance of diabetic foot care by washing, drying, and assessing feet daily for sores." The goal must also be achievable. In the example of diabetic foot care, an obese client who cannot reach his feet may not be able to wash and dry his feet himself. This client may need a care plan that calls for a caregiver to clean and assess his feet.

> 🔍 A common tool used by case managers when creating a care plan is the acronym SMART. The care plan goals must be **S**pecific to the client, **M**easurable, **A**chievable, **R**ealistic, and **T**ime-Oriented.

IMPLEMENTATION

The **implementation** step of case management involves taking the necessary action to complete the prescribed goals. This may include care coordination to ensure the client's interdisciplinary team is on the same page. The CCM may also clarify medication directions, schedule appointments, research financial resources, obtain medical equipment, and explain lab reports to the client.

Following Up

Following up with the client is necessary to determine the effectiveness of the implementation step. Scheduling a doctor's appointment is worthless if the client does not go to the appointment. The client's need for a change in the care plan strategy is evaluated in this step. The following-up stage of case management is ensuring that the client understands and is completing their goals. This process is continually evolving and being revised until the CCM and client are satisfied.

Transitioning

When a patient is discharged from a health care facility such as a hospital, skilled nursing home, or rehab center, the patient is **transitioning**. Transitioning may be from one health care setting to another or to the patient's home. The transitioning phase of patient care is an important one for the CCM. There is a potential for miscommunication and even harm to the patient during this phase. The CCM steps in and assists the patient with important education and care coordination to achieve the goal of relocating safely to another setting.

Post-Transition Communication

When being discharged from a health care setting to the home, discharge paperwork will be given to the patient. This includes vital information such as changes in medication status. The CCM will complete medication reconciliation and prevent a potential hospital readmission. **Post-transitioning communication** with the prescribing physician for medication clarification is frequently needed. Continuity of care is important in the post-transition phase. This will include ensuring the patient has scheduled the requested follow-up doctor appointments. Physical therapy, home health nurses, and a home health aide for grooming needs may be requested by the physician. Post-transitioning communication is required for the CCM to ensure all these important needs are fulfilled.

> Polypharmacy is the practice of administering multiple medications concurrently. The elderly are the highest population for polypharmacy and are at the greatest risk for accidental misuse. CCMs can help the elderly population by assisting with education and medication management.

Evaluation

Did the client achieve their goals to improve their health? It is time to find out in the **evaluation** phase of case management. All problems listed on the care plan will at some time need evaluation. The goals on the care plan may be either subjective or objective. To achieve an **objective goal**, the CCM will be able to witness the achievement. There will be physical evidence of reaching the goal. For example, to evaluate a blood pressure goal, the CCM may observe the values from actually checking blood pressure with a monitor. A **subjective goal** is not witnessed by the CCM but rather is voiced by the client. In this case, the client may tell the CCM what the blood pressure reading was when she checked it. To effectively evaluate if your client's blood pressure goals have been met, objective goals are advised.

2. The CCM calls the client's doctor to ask if a fax was received from the pharmacist regarding a medication discrepancy on the hospital discharge summary. This is an example of which phase in the case management process?

A) planning

B) assessing

C) evaluation

D) following up

3. The client had routine labs drawn, and his goal is to achieve an A1C value of 6. The lab value was 7, so the goal was not achieved. What type of goal is this?

A) subjective

B) compliant

C) objective

D) mandated

The Role of Case Managers in Different Settings

Case managers are fortunate to be able to showcase their skills in a variety of settings. Although each setting may require the case manager to take on different roles, ensuring the client is functioning as well as possible is always the main goal. This section focuses on a variety of settings and the unique responsibilities in each setting.

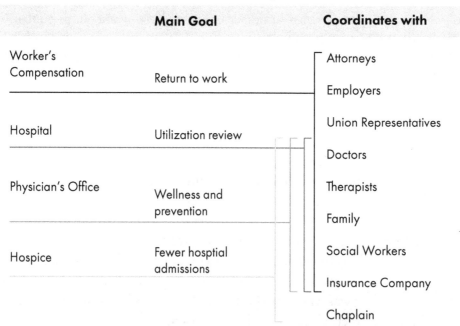

	Main Goal	Coordinates with
Worker's Compensation	Return to work	Attorneys
		Employers
Hospital	Utilization review	Union Representatives
		Doctors
Physician's Office	Wellness and prevention	Therapists
		Family
Hospice	Fewer hosptial admissions	Social Workers
		Insurance Company
		Chaplain

Figure 1.1. Role of the Case Manager

A **hospital case manager** will focus on **discharge planning**. Where will the patient be going when she leaves the hospital? Will she have all the tools she needs to be safe and in optimum health at the new residence? Continuity of care is a priority and ensures there are no gaps in care.

Hospital case managers may also be trained in **utilization management**. This is a process that reviews services while the patient is in the hospital. In this clerical role, the CCM determines if the patient is in the appropriate setting with the highest level of quality care. The case manager will review the services ordered by physicians and determine if the services are medically necessary.

A case manager in a **physician's office** setting is focused on prevention of health-related concerns. Reminding the patient about wellness exams and assisting with scheduling the exam are duties this case manager may perform. Ensuring that the patient is educated on the doctor's instructions and medication orders is another task this case manager will face.

Palliative and **hospice care organizations** hire case managers as well. These case managers are unique in the aspect that they also provide hands-on, direct patient care. Frequent communication with the physician for medication instruction is part of this role, as the stages of the dying process advance. Often the patient is not able to communicate at this point, and a patient advocate is needed. The case manager will shine in this role.

Workers' Compensation case management is a growing field. The employer and employee wish to have the employee return to work as soon as possible after a work-related injury or illness. Coordination of care is still a priority in this setting; however, the communication involves additional professionals such as attorneys and claim adjusters.

PRACTICE QUESTION

4. What is the primary goal of a CCM in a physician office setting?

A) discharge planning

B) prevention of medical concerns

C) communication with the client's employer

D) utilization management

Answer Key

1. A) Incorrect. The CCM wants to ensure the patient is not at risk for readmission to the hospital and has all the correct medications.
   B) Incorrect. The CCM's goal is to ensure the patient has the optimum level of care.
   C) **Correct.** Although the patient is supposed to rest, the CCM should promote autonomy and self-advocacy. The CCM should encourage the patient to play an active role in their health care management.
   D) Incorrect. The CCM wishes to lower health care costs.

2. A) Incorrect. The CCM is not planning.
   B) Incorrect. This is not the assessing phase.
   C) Incorrect. This action is not part of the evaluation phase.
   D) **Correct.** The CCM followed up with the physician to resolve a gap in care.

3. A) Incorrect. This goal was not strictly perceived by the patient.
   B) Incorrect. This is not a goal of compliance.
   C) **Correct.** This goal was evidenced by lab values.
   D) Incorrect. This goal was not mandated.

4. A) Incorrect. A CCM working in a hospital focuses on discharge planning.
   B) **Correct.** Prevention of medical concerns is a primary focus for a physician office CCM.
   C) Incorrect. Communicating with the employer is a role of a Workers' Compensation CCM.
   D) Incorrect. Utilization management is more specific to a CCM working in a hospital.

TWO: CARE DELIVERY

Continuum of Care

Continuum of care can be defined as the comprehensive monitoring and tracking of a client and his or her care through all disciplines and stages of health care. When looking at the continuum of care, the case manager must consider:

+ where and how care began

+ where and how care ended

+ which discipline was responsible for a client's care at each stage of transition

Consider a fifty-eight-year-old post-CVA client with left-sided paralysis who is being discharged from the hospital to home care with orders for physical therapy, occupational therapy, and speech therapy. In order to manage the discharge and next steps for the client, the case manager must be familiar with each stage of the client's hospitalization, the multidisciplinary personnel at each stage, the reason for the consult of each discipline, and that discipline's findings and recommendations.

Continuum of care works by establishing a comprehensive storyline of the client's care: from incident and chief complaint through assessment, diagnosis, planning, implementation, and evaluation of care. During this process, the client's providers are kept well informed of changes and new developments in the client's plan of care. The continuum of care can be thought of as a relay race in which each runner hands the same baton to another member of his or her team. Think of the baton as the client's chart, and each member of the team as another medical discipline.

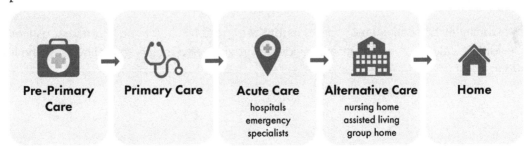

Pre-Primary Care → **Primary Care** → **Acute Care** hospitals emergency specialists → **Alternative Care** nursing home assisted living group home → **Home**

Figure 2.1. Continuum of Care

The case manager may be involved during some or all of a client's continuum of care. The case manager may initially be responsible only for performing a **utilization review** to determine medical necessity of a hospital visit or stay.

During a client's time in the hospital, the certified case manager (CCM) may need to perform a **concurrent review** to determine if the appropriate level of care is being provided. The CCM will visit the client and/or caregiver while the client is hospitalized and review the relevant medical history to determine if continued admission to the hospital is warranted.

If the CCM is also coordinating care, they may get in touch with the client's primary care provider and other specialists involved in the client's care to review the plan of care and next steps of treatment.

When it comes time to discharge or transition a client to either home or a lower level of care, the case manager wears the hat of the discharge planner. At that point, it is the case manager's responsibility to ensure that:

1. the client has completed all necessary testing/procedures that have been ordered or that he or she has consented to.

2. the primary attending provider and other disciplines have signed off on the discharge or transfer.

3. the discharge/transfer paperwork was explained to the client, and the client understood what was explained to him or her (generally indicated by the client's signature).

4. follow-up appointments and medication information are included on discharge summary.

5. the client is transitioned to the appropriate level of care.

6. the client has a safe place to be discharged to and a support system in place.

7. there are no barriers to discharge (e.g., lack of place to be discharged to, lack of pharmacy access, etc.).

8. the client knows warning signs to monitor to prevent readmission.

Many federally and state-operated managed-care organizations (such as Medicare and Medicaid) rely on case managers to facilitate the continuum of care for the underserved population of these agencies, and that may start with the care of the homeless and/or indigent. Those clients must be followed through state-funded health care facilities to their ultimate destination: a loved one's home, a halfway house, or a shelter. From that point, it is the case manager's responsibility to ensure that clients have access to the resources they need to continue self-management of their health.

> Continuity or continuum of care is essential to a client's health care process, as it establishes a smooth transition from provider to provider and facility to facility (or to the home environment).

PRACTICE QUESTION

1. When considering discharge or transitional care planning for a client, the case manager should be familiar with all the following EXCEPT:

    A) the client's admission diagnosis

    B) the client's treatment plan

    C) other disciplines consulting on the client's case

    D) the client's initial stage of hospitalization only

Levels of Care and Care Settings

There are several levels of care to which a client can and may be transitioned. **Acute care** involves immediate, short-term care for illness or trauma. Acute care can be delivered in a hospital or nursing unit, emergency department, or urgent care facility.

Subacute care is for patients who are medically stable but require short-term inpatient care or therapy. These clients may have an acute illness or injury, may be experiencing a worsening of a chronic condition, or may be recovering from surgery. Subacute care can be given in a hospital step-down unit, rehabilitation facility, or skilled nursing facility, provided that the client is medically stable for this transition.

> Patients who may require subacute care include those diagnosed with closed-head injuries, spinal injuries, or strokes; patients recovering from surgery; patients who require frequent assessment; and patients prescribed IV antibiotics.

Transitional care is care provided during transition from one facility to another (such as a hospital to a nursing home, or a skilled nursing facility to the client's home). **Ambulatory care** primarily involves a client taking him- or herself to a facility to be treated for an illness or injury and is usually administered in an outpatient setting, such as a clinic, an urgent care facility, a free-standing emergency department, or a physician's office.

PRACTICE QUESTION

2. A patient has been admitted to the intensive care unit after a heart attack. What level of care is the patient receiving?

    A) acute care

    B) subacute care

    C) transitional care

    D) ambulatory care

Alternative Care Facilities

Many facilities fall under the description of *alternative care*. A **nursing home** provides care to those clients who have suffered a health-altering event (such as a CVA or heart attack) and who also require much assistance with activities of daily living (ADLs).

An **assisted living facility** is similar to a residential development but is designed for mostly independent adults who need assistance with activities of daily living (such as walking, eating, toileting, etc.) but do not require care in a nursing home. These individuals may have experienced an acute injury or illness (such as a minor stroke or heart attack) or be chronically ill with conditions such as diabetes or chronic obstructive pulmonary disease (COPD).

Group homes are living facilities for people requiring care or constant observation. Examples of group homes include those that assist individuals with disabilities, and those that provide shelter to children or teenage victims of abuse. Most often, a social worker and a therapist will work in a group home to provide emotional support and care to the individuals residing there.

A **residential treatment facility** is one in which the primary focus is to assist individuals who have substance abuse issues with treating and overcoming their addictions. The staff of a residential treatment facility will include doctors, nurses, psychiatrists, and counselors.

PRACTICE QUESTION

3.   Mary is a sixty-eight-year-old female who was mentally sound and capable of performing activities of daily living until she suffered a severe stroke one year ago. Mary is now unable to feed or dress herself and requires assistance with toileting and bathing. At which facility will she most likely receive the care she needs?

   A)   assisted living facility

   B)   nursing home

   C)   group home

   D)   residential treatment facility

Health Care Providers

In today's society, with a considerable amount of educational opportunities and options and innovative technological advances, there exists a never-ending variety of health care providers from which to choose. **Physicians** include general (family) practitioners and specialists. Physicians spend many years in medical school and training to earn a degree in medicine, then they must take certification exams to legally practice medicine. They can diagnose conditions, order procedures, treat and write medication prescriptions for illnesses, and they will usually see a client in their office.

Physician assistants (PAs) assist a physician and can basically operate within the same scope of practice as a physician but with limitations contingent on their education and professional experience, state regulations, office policies and procedures, and clients' needs. They may collect a comprehensive medical history, perform a physical head-to-toe assessment, diagnose illnesses, prescribe medications, and establish care plans.

Nurse practitioners (NPs) possess a master's degree or higher in nursing and function in a similar capacity to that of a physician. They may diagnose and treat illnesses and also write prescriptions.

Clinical nurse specialists (CNSs) have advanced education and training in a specialized field, such as psychiatric care, women's health, or critical care. CNSs have attended and graduated from an accredited school of nursing, possess a master's or doctoral degree in nursing, and have passed a specialized certification exam. They can make diagnoses, develop treatment plans, and provide care; they are also often in leadership roles where they supervise other nurses.

Registered nurses (RNs) and **licensed vocational/practical nurses (LVNs/LPNs)** typically do not have advanced degrees. They will carry out orders from a physician, physician's assistant, or nurse practitioner; collect medical histories; perform assessments; develop a nursing diagnosis and treatment plan; implement the treatment plan; and evaluate clients' outcomes.

Nurse technicians provide care for patients under the supervision of an RN or other more credentialed health care providers. There is no official certification or scope of practice for nurse technicians, but some nursing coursework is usually required. Nursing techs are often students working toward a nursing degree or recent graduates looking to gain work experience.

Behavioral health care providers dedicate their lives to supporting and preserving the mental/emotional health and well-being of mentally ill individuals. A **psychiatrist** is a physician who has attended medical school, obtained a degree in medicine, and chosen to specialize in psychiatry. These physicians can write prescriptions for anti-anxiety medications and anti-depressants, among other medications.

Psychiatrists are not to be confused with **psychologists**, who must undergo training and an internship to secure an advanced degree in psychology. While psychologists may have a doctoral degree, they are not medical doctors and therefore cannot prescribe medications. They offer focused counseling services that can assist in the diagnosis and treatment of medical and emotional issues.

Licensed professional counselors (LPCs) possess a master's or doctoral degree in counseling and will, within their scope of practice, offer collaborative, therapeutic counseling to those individuals who seek professional guidance to promote emotional, behavioral, and mental health and well-being.

Licensed clinical social workers (LCSWs) are licensed to practice in a clinical or counseling setting and directly intermingle with clients to diagnose and treat mental, emotional, and behavioral issues. LCSWs will also often focus on public health and develop/implement new and advanced measures to facilitate and promote communication within the community.

Community vendors provide goods and services to the whole of a community. One such example is a **community health fair**. During the fair, health care professionals will talk to individuals about their health and ways to promote a healthy lifestyle. They will also often record vital signs and weight. Another type of community vendor would be a **community-based day program**. Community-based day programs include after-school activities for children and outpatient behavioral management programs. Alcoholics Anonymous (AA) and Narcotics Anonymous (NA) are well-known examples of community-based programs. They offer emotional support and guidance to those living in recovery from addiction.

> 🔍 While the overarching goal of all health care providers is to promote a healthy lifestyle and healthy outcomes, each provider's scope of practice is very different. Case managers should help the client decide which medical professional is appropriate to meet their needs.

PRACTICE QUESTION

4. Which of the following health care providers can prescribe medication?

- **A)** psychologists
- **B)** nurse practitioners
- **C)** registered nurses
- **D)** licensed professional counselors

Interdisciplinary Care Team (ICT)

The **interdisciplinary care team (ICT)** comprises health care providers from different fields who work together to provide care for the patient. The members of a client's ICT largely depend on the client's chief complaint, diagnosis, and treatment goals. In general, the ICT will include a primary care physician, the attending physician (if the client is in the hospital), a case manager, and other consulting health care personnel, including physicians, nurses, and therapists with relevant specialties. The ICT may also include social workers, chaplains, dieticians, or pharmacists.

Each individual on the team has specific tasks. The client's physician is responsible for diagnosing and treating his or her illness or injury but may also refer the client to consulting specialists or occupational health professionals. Those individuals will speak with the physician about the client, see the client for assessment, and make a recommendation to the physician based on assessment findings and test results. A client may have many specialists consulting on his or her case. The case manager will review the client's medical record, physician's documentation, test results, care plan, and consulting specialists' assessments and recommendations. The case manager may get in touch with the physician to discuss treatment options and transitions to another level of care.

The responsibilities of each member of the ICT ultimately and optimally culminate into one central objective: to develop a comprehensive plan of care that addresses each team member's measurable and attainable goals for the client.

There is a distinct difference between the terms *interdisciplinary* and *multidisciplinary*. Interdisciplinary care focuses on the formulation of a collective care plan, to which each member of the ICT can contribute. Multidisciplinary care does not stress a unified approach to care. Instead, each team member utilizes his or her own specialized skills and capabilities to establish separate care goals.

PRACTICE QUESTION

5. Within the interdisciplinary care team (ICT), the role of the case manager is to
   A) make a diagnosis.
   B) refer the client to a specialist.
   C) coordinate care.
   D) provide emotional counseling.

Client Assessment
PHYSICAL FUNCTIONING

A **physical functioning assessment** will evaluate a client's level of physical functioning with regard to his or her ability to perform activities of daily living and instrumental activities of daily living. **Activities of daily living (ADLs)** are those activities an individual must accomplish to arise in the morning, move from place to place, and finish up the day. They include walking, brushing teeth, toileting, bathing, dressing, and eating. **Instrumental activities of daily living (IADLs)** involve activities that an individual can perform after they have arisen in the morning and are up, ready to face the day. These activities include cooking, driving, using the telephone/computer, shopping, bookkeeping, and managing medications.

A physical functioning assessment provides health care professionals with information about the client's activity limitations in their environment. It addresses:

+ lower and upper extremity mobility
+ elimination habits with emphasis on continence
+ oral and dental health
+ visual, auditory, olfactory, sensory, and gustatory health
+ the ability to lift a specific pound or kilogram weight
+ manual dexterity and coordination
+ environmental barriers to safety (stairs, loose carpeting, exposed wires)
+ sensitivity to extremes of temperature and moisture

This information is used to determine the safety of a client's environment, the risk of falls or fractures, the risk of disability and depression, the requirement of other therapies (such as speech, physical, and occupational), anticipated additional health care needs, and the quality of life the client will have as the result of a limitation.

> 🔍 It is a common misconception that physical functioning assessments are mainly used to determine the physical abilities or limitations of the elderly. They can also be employed to evaluate children with special needs and persons with disabilities.

PRACTICE QUESTION

6. Which of the following is an instrumental activity of daily living?

A) bathing

B) toileting

C) eating

D) cooking

BEHAVIORAL HEALTH ASSESSMENTS

Information about a client's behavior can be gathered by requesting that he or she complete a patient health questionnaire, such as the one shown in Figure 2.2. These questionnaires can help providers screen for issues such as depression, generalized anxiety disorder, and alcohol dependence. This data is instrumental in identifying emotional and mental health needs, the possible requirement of a referral to a mental or behavioral health care professional, and barriers to compliance with a treatment plan. It also assists in recognizing a client's access to a support system.

A **behavioral health assessment** (or mental health assessment) focuses on evaluating an individual's behavior within a setting where he or she may be more likely to exhibit difficulty in controlling his or her behavior. The assessment is a valuable tool for the physician or psychiatrist to diagnose and treat mental illness. This is important for clients who may be depressed and wish to harm themselves or others.

There are two types of behavioral/mental health assessments: clinical and functional. A **clinical behavioral assessment** centers on the behavior displayed by an individual in the home environment, at work, or at school, and the similarities in behavior in each setting. After an evaluation of the findings, the assessor can formulate a concise plan of care for review by the individual's other health care providers.

A **functional behavioral assessment** explores the reasons for unsuitable behaviors. It is designed to identify the cause behind specific behaviors so the cause itself (and not just the behavior) can be addressed.

Behavioral health assessments are performed by qualified mental health professionals. However, the CCM may report their observations of the client to medical professionals and participate in the formulation of the care plan.

The CCM will also play a critical role in ensuring that the client adheres to the treatment plan that results from the behavioral assessment. The CCM may review the physician's treatment plan and medications prescribed and may assess the client to ensure there is compliance with medication administration. If noncompliance with medication administration is noted, the CCM may pursue the reasoning behind the noncompliance and assist the client with resolving the issues.

Personal Health Questionnaire Depression Scale (PHQ–8)

Over the last **two weeks**, how often have you been bothered by any of the following problems? (circle **one number** on each line)

How often during the past 2 weeks were you bothered by...	Not at all	Several days	More than half the days	Nearly every day
1. Little interest or pleasure in doing things	0	1	2	3
2. Feeling down, depressed, or hopeless	0	1	2	3
3. Trouble falling or staying asleep, or sleeping too much	0	1	2	3
4. Feeling tired or having little energy	0	1	2	3
5. Poor appetite or overeating	0	1	2	3
6. Feeling bad about yourself, or that you are a failure, or have let yourself or your family down	0	1	2	3
7. Trouble concentrating on things such as reading the newspaper or watching television	0	1	2	3
8. Moving or speaking so slowly that other people could have noticed; or the opposite—being so fidgety or restless that that you have been moving around a lot more than usual	0	1	2	3

Figure 2.2. Example of a Patient Health Questionnaire

PRACTICE QUESTION

7. You are the case manager for a seven-year-old client whose mother reports that he has been acting out, cursing, and throwing tantrums at home, at school, and in public. Which type of behavioral assessment will most likely be conducted?

    A) clinical

    B) functional

    C) mental

    D) emotional

Client's Acuity and Severity Levels

Acuity in the medical community refers to the level of severity or complexity of an illness or injury. Many factors can determine a client's acuity level, such as:

+ acute/chronic illness
+ chief complaint
+ status following a procedure or surgery

+ receiving blood or blood products
+ risk of harm to self/others
+ physical functional status
+ mental/behavioral status

Typically, a nurse caring for higher-acuity clients will have fewer clients, while a nurse who has basic lower-level–acuity clients will have more. This is generally true for case management as well. The case manager will manage their caseload in accordance with who was most recently discharged from the hospital, who is presenting with new onset of symptoms, who is having difficulty with self-management of condition, and so on.

In some settings, the case manager may be given a set number of cases regardless of acuity level. For example, insurance companies hire case managers who are assigned a certain number of cases regardless of acuity level. In this example, the insurance CCM sees clients based on their assigned territory and proximity to their home.

InterQual and Milliman Care Guidelines (MCG) are two evidence-based solutions that assist physicians, nurses, and other health care professionals with making decisions about client acuity, appropriate level of care, and staffing. They each contain levels of care criteria and guidelines to direct client care. **InterQual** uses an algorithm flow process to determine next steps in treatment. For example, if a patient presents to the emergency department with abdominal pain, the first question may be about onset of pain (acute or chronic). The answer to that question will lead to another asking whether the client is appropriate for observation care or admission. With this type of system, health care professionals and especially case managers can determine appropriate care rather quickly.

Milliman Care Guidelines (MCG) offer a quick search option for signs and symptoms, and then the user is taken to every listing with those signs and symptoms. One click will direct the user to care planning options, clinical indications for admission, alternatives to hospitalization, and discharge possibilities. These are both useful tools in making decisions about appropriate levels of care, acuity, and staffing.

PRACTICE QUESTION

8. Blanca is the charge nurse for the medical-surgical unit and is making assignments for the oncoming shift. For nursing care, she knows that the higher the acuity level, the

A) higher the nurse-to-client ratio.

B) higher the physician-to-client ratio.

C) lower the nurse-to-client ratio.

D) lower the physician-to-client ratio.

Adherence to Care Regimen

Adherence, in reference to a care or treatment plan, means that the client is complying with physician-recommended treatments and heeding medical advice. **Nonadherence** (also known as noncompliance) means that the client is not complying with physician recommendations. A client may be noncompliant with a treatment plan for a variety of reasons. He or she may not agree with what has been recommended, or barriers may exist that would impede compliance. Such barriers include finances, educational status, sensory deficits, and language/culture/ethnicity. Consequences of noncompliance can include exacerbation of an existing condition, development of an acute condition, or death.

Before any treatment plan is executed, it is essential to assess a client's readiness and willingness to change certain behaviors. After that has been established, every member of a client's health care team must ensure that the client comprehends what is expected of him or her. Some health care professionals believe in the "tough love" approach when caring for a noncompliant client, meaning that worst-case scenarios are discussed in detail to inspire the client to make necessary lifestyle changes; however, no matter what, the client will change when he or she wants to and is ready to.

Educating clients is key in helping them reach their health goals, so an explanation of what is going on with their bodies concerning a particular health condition will go a long way in promoting and maintaining adherence to a treatment plan. Encouraging questions and feedback is also instrumental in achieving this goal. Including a client in the decision-making process and collaborating with him or her during each step of treatment will help as well. Health care professionals should act as coaches walking alongside clients as they navigate the road to healthy outcomes and better quality of life.

PRACTICE QUESTION

9. All of the following could be consequences of noncompliance with a treatment plan EXCEPT:

   A) improvement of a condition

   B) worsening of a condition

   C) development of an acute condition

   D) death

Management of Clients

CLIENTS WITH ACUTE ILLNESS

The management of a client with an acute illness comes with many challenges. When working with a client with an acute illness, the duties of the nurse case manager focus on:

- stabilization of the client
- thorough assessment
- collaboration with the client's attending physician or primary care physician
- consistent monitoring
- development of a care or treatment plan
- discharge planning

A client with an acute illness has typically been admitted to a hospital with a new diagnosis. The CCM will be educating this client about the new illness and what prevention measures to take. High readmission potential is a concern if the proper acute illness treatment plan is not understood. The CCM will also assist with scheduling all follow-up medical appointments, as well as researching transportation needs to the appointments. Any new medical equipment prescribed may be obtained with the CCM's assistance.

The CCM must ensure the client is taking the correct medications prescribed by the hospital attending physician. This is usually done by performing a medication reconciliation. Medications in the client's home are compared to the medication discharge summary paperwork. Any discrepancies noted are addressed with the client and the prescribing physician, if necessary.

The **complementary nursing** acute care model was developed to promote continuity of care by one nurse throughout a client's acute illness, from onset to prehospital state. The model reduces health care costs, improves health care quality, improves the coordination of care, promotes the expansion of nursing knowledge, and prevents readmissions. In today's ever-changing and fast-paced health care environment, we are increasingly beginning to embrace a "one-stop shop" care model that concentrates on one or two health care professionals throughout the care continuum who are proficient in numerous areas, instead of many specialized individuals. However, even when this model is used, clients often see numerous specialists, requiring committed care coordination from the case manager.

PRACTICE QUESTION

10. The purpose of the complementary nursing care model is to do all of the following EXCEPT

    A) decrease the client's health care costs

    B) improve care coordination for the client

    C) prevent readmission of the client to the hospital

    D) increase the number of providers the client sees

CLIENTS WITH CHRONIC ILLNESS

The responsibilities of caring for a client with a chronic illness are complex, especially if the client suffers from more than one illness. A detailed health history must be completed, which includes (but is not limited to) main diagnosis, names and specialties of all providers, list of current medications, and hospitalization and surgery history. Additionally, a case manager working with a client with a chronic illness, must:

+ collaborate with the interdisciplinary care team
+ review/update the treatment plan as necessary
+ educate the client about the disease process
+ identify barriers to compliance and access to care
+ anticipate possible post-discharge complications

Education is an important part of the CCM job description for chronically ill clients. The CCM must ensure their client understands their medication administration and regime. For example, the CCM may have the client demonstrate the proper way to use their breathing machine. A thorough educational plan will help the client better manage their chronic illness.

PRACTICE QUESTION

11. Care coordination for the chronically ill client would rely heavily upon all of the following EXCEPT

A) collaboration among interdisciplinary and multidisciplinary care teams

B) identifying barriers to access to care

C) anticipation of possible post-discharge complications

D) maintaining the same treatment plan throughout care

HOSPICE, PALLIATIVE, AND END-OF-LIFE CARE

Caring for a client in hospice, palliative care, or at the end of life can be challenging. Health care professionals must provide emotional support to the client and the family, while making the client as comfortable as possible through pain and symptom management and relaxation techniques. Health care for these clients is very different from other types of care. Case managers and other health care personnel will eventually lose these clients to the disease or condition that brought them to hospice or end-of-life care in the first place. This can be difficult to witness and comprehend.

Building a trusting rapport with the client and his or her family is a key factor when providing care. Some health care professionals almost become part of the family. Case managers must remain cognizant of the client's and family's cultural and spiritual beliefs during this time and respect those as much as possible. Ethical dilemmas are often discussed when determining what is right, fair, and, most importantly, what most closely aligns with the client's wishes. A case manager takes all this into consideration while focusing on a review of the treatment plan, updating changes in medications, and assisting the client and his or her family through the grieving and death processes.

12. A case manager has just taken on a new client with stage IV colon cancer. The client's family is struggling to process end-of-life issues. What can the CCM do initially to attempt to ease the family's suffering?

- **A)** introduce himself to the family and then leave quickly, allowing them to grieve privately
- **B)** introduce himself to the family and begin talking to them about the client's medications and treatment plan
- **C)** introduce himself to the family, sit down, and ask about the client's medical history
- **D)** introduce himself to the family, sit down, and begin a conversation with the client's family about the client's life

CLIENTS WITH DISABILITIES

A **disability** can be defined as a physical, mental, or sensory deficit that may impair one's ability to perform ADLs and/or interact with others. One must tread carefully when caring for a client with a disability; although they are disabled, there are still plenty of things they *can* do, so the CCM should focus on that fact and be sensitive to it. Allowing a client to demonstrate his or her capabilities promotes independence and boosts self-esteem.

Specific goals are key in caring for a client with disabilities. For example, when completing the physical functioning assessment, the responsible health care professional must consider physical capabilities and limitations and then develop a goal-oriented treatment plan to address said limitations. Part of this assessment should include an **environmental evaluation**, which is designed to determine how the client interacts within his or her environment, and whether the environment is a hindrance or a help to the client.

 A case manager should keep in close contact with durable medical equipment companies to ensure that clients with disabilities have everything they need to function.

A mental/emotional health assessment is also vital to the complete care of the individual. The client's feelings about their disability will greatly affect how they cope with it and how receptive they are to change certain behaviors that may improve the quality of life with the disability.

Often other health care disciplines will be involved (such as physical, speech, and occupational therapists), resulting in a complex health care plan. When this happens, the case manager may need to explain these complexities to the client in a format they can understand.

PRACTICE QUESTION

13. When caring for an individual with disabilities, what is a case manager's primary focus?

   A) assessing the client's capabilities

   B) environmental access

   C) ensuring that the client can perform activities for daily living

   D) providing access to occupational therapy

CLIENTS WITH MULTIPLE CHRONIC ILLNESSES

Case management of clients with multiple chronic illnesses is complex because there are many different conditions to treat. Additionally, patients usually have several specialists and have been prescribed a long list of medications. Caring for these clients differs from caring for clients with a singular chronic illness, in that the case manager must collaborate not only with the ICT but also with the multidisciplinary care team. Furthermore, each health care specialty will have its own individual set of measurable goals for the client, and the case manager must integrate these into the treatment plan to ensure that all issues are addressed. Discharge planning can be challenging for the case manager, as each specialty or consult must sign off on discharge orders, and upon discharge, the case manager must educate the client about each condition and treatment goals and ensure that he or she understands.

PRACTICE QUESTION

14. A case manager caring for an individual with multiple chronic illnesses must consider his or her role in which of the following?

   A) educating the client about one specific chronic condition

   B) ensuring that the client has the necessary durable medical equipment to manage one condition

   C) collaboration with other disciplines that focuses on more than one condition

   D) development of a treatment plan that addresses a single, but serious, illness

TRANSITIONS OF CARE AND TRANSITIONAL CARE

Transition of care is best described as the care provided for a client as he or she is transitioned from one level of care to another. The case manager will perform intake, complete an assessment, collaborate with the client's physician(s) to develop a treatment plan and coordinate care, ensure that the next level of care is appropriate for the client, plan discharge, and perform follow-up with the client. The case manager will essentially follow the client through the stages of care, while updating the treatment plan along the way. One of the main duties of the care manager in this capacity is to ensure that each transition is as smooth as possible, and that everyone involved at each stage is well informed of the client's condition and status.

PRACTICE QUESTION

15. Which responsibility does NOT fall under the scope of responsibility of the case manager when transitioning a client from one level of care to another?

   A) client follow-up

   B) discharge planning

   C) care coordination

   D) appeal reviewer

MEDICATION THERAPY MANAGEMENT AND RECONCILIATION

Medication reconciliation has become increasingly important over the last two decades. **Medication reconciliation** is the process of reviewing the name, dosage, route, frequency, and reason for each medication at each level of care. It is also three-pronged; the process is reviewed from the physician to the client and the client's caregiver. Within multiple care level transitions, medication information can be lost or misplaced, so review must take place after every transition. The process itself involves:

   + Obtaining a thorough list of current administered medications from the client or caregiver, complete with:

      ✧ medication name,   ✧ frequency, and

      ✧ dosage,   ✧ purpose.

      ✧ route,

   + Complete transmission of that information to admission history, transfer and discharge paperwork.

   + Comparing that information to the received transfer or discharge paperwork to ensure that it is complete and to identify any inconsistencies. Such differences would need to be brought to the attention of the entire health care team, and changes to the orders would have to be made.

PRACTICE QUESTION

16. Which of the following is NOT part of medication reconciliation?

   A) medication expiration date

   B) medication name

   C) medication frequency

   D) medication purpose

Answer Key

1. A) Incorrect. The case manager can and will review the admission diagnosis, as well as any other diagnoses that are made throughout the health care continuum.

    B) Incorrect. The case manager can and will continually review/update the client's treatment plan.

    C) Incorrect. The case manager is aware of and has reviewed all consults on the client's case, as well as their findings and recommendations.

    D) Correct. The case manager will have thorough knowledge of each stage of the client's care.

2. **A) Correct.** The intensive care unit provides short-term inpatient care for patients with acute illness or injury.

3. A) Incorrect. An assisted living facility is for independent adults who need minimal assistance with activities of daily living.

    B) Correct. A nursing home would be the best option for this client, as she needs a lot of help with feeding, dressing, toileting, and bathing herself.

    C) Incorrect. A group home is more appropriate for individuals who require a lot of care and supervision but who are somewhat independent.

    D) Incorrect. A residential treatment facility is the best choice for individuals who are trying to overcome substance abuse or addiction.

4. **B) Correct.** A nurse practitioner can prescribe medication. Psychologists, registered nurses, and licensed professional counselors cannot.

5. A) Incorrect. The attending physician or a specialist provider will make a diagnosis.

    B) Incorrect. The attending physician will refer clients to specialists for further assessment.

    C) Correct. The case manager ensures continuity of care between all providers.

    D) Incorrect. While the case manager may provide emotional support, the ICT should include licensed mental health professionals to provide counseling.

6. **D) Correct.** Cooking is considered an instrumental activity of daily living, as it is not associated with necessary functioning throughout the day. The other choices are activities of daily living.

7. **A) Correct.** A clinical behavioral assessment will be conducted on this client, as he is exhibiting similar inappropriate behaviors in more than one setting.

    B) Incorrect. A functional behavioral assessment is typically used to explore the causes for a specific behavior.

C) Incorrect. A mental health assessment is sometimes used interchangeably with a behavioral health assessment but differs from a clinical behavioral health assessment.

D) Incorrect. An emotional health assessment would not be appropriate at this time but may serve to determine additional treatment options in the future.

8. A) Incorrect. If client acuity is high, the nurse most likely will not have many clients to care for.

B) Incorrect. Ratio of physician to client is not relevant when discussing nursing and case management.

C) Correct. If client acuity is high, the nurse will have fewer clients to care for.

D) Incorrect. Ratio of physician to client is not relevant when discussing nursing and case management.

9. **A) Correct.** Condition improvement is not likely in the face of treatment plan noncompliance.

B) Incorrect. Worsening or exacerbation of a chronic condition will almost always happen during noncompliance.

C) Incorrect. The development of an acute condition can sometimes happen when a client is noncompliant with a treatment plan.

D) Incorrect. Death can sometimes be a consequence of noncompliance with a treatment plan.

10. A) Incorrect. Complementary nursing supports decreased health care costs.

B) Incorrect. Complementary nursing results in an improvement in care coordination.

C) Incorrect. Complementary nursing prevents readmissions.

D) Correct. In the complementary nursing care model, care is administered by fewer providers instead of many specialized ones.

11. A) Incorrect. Collaboration within ICT and MCT is essential in caring for chronically ill clients, as each team has valuable input about how to best manage client care.

B) Incorrect. Identification of barriers to access to care must be done to assess readiness for self-management and discharge.

C) Incorrect. The nurse case manager will anticipate possible post-discharge complications while the client is still under his or her care to determine the need for additional care options.

D) Correct. Throughout stages and transitions of care, a chronically ill client's care plan will change and evolve.

12. A) Incorrect. Sometimes leaving is the best option, but in this case, the family needs to be supported and comforted.

B) Incorrect. Having a clinical discussion with the family will make the nurse seem cold and distant, which is not what the family needs at this time.

C) Incorrect. Asking questions about the client's medical history is not appropriate, as the nurse should have already reviewed the client's chart.

D) **Correct.** Starting a discussion of the client's life will facilitate the building of trust, and this will help the family open up and begin to come to terms with what is happening.

13. **A)** **Correct.** Before assessing what a client cannot do because of disability, it is important to evaluate what the client can do. Knowing this information will guide the goals of the care plan.

B) Incorrect. Determining whether a disabled client can access necessities in their environment will be part of the physical functioning assessment, but it will not be the primary focus.

C) Incorrect. Ensuring that the disabled client has everything he or she needs to accomplish ADL is imperative, but those needs will most likely be assessed at another time.

D) Incorrect. As with performing ADLs, the need for other health care disciplines will be addressed at another time.

14. A) Incorrect. A case manager will educate the client about all his or her chronic conditions, not just one.

B) Incorrect. While this is essential, the case manager will ensure that the client has the necessary tools and equipment to manage all conditions.

C) **Correct.** A case manager will collaborate with many health care disciplines on behalf of the client to guarantee that the care plan is comprehensive and that all disciplines have had an opportunity for input.

D) Incorrect. The care plan for the client with multiple chronic illnesses will address goals of the treatment of all chronic conditions, not just one.

15. **D)** **Correct.** The case manager will not function in the role of an appeal reviewer when transitioning a client. All the other choices are responsibilities of the case manager.

16. **A)** **Correct.** Medication expiration date is not typically included in medication reconciliation. The other choices are all part of medication reconciliation.

THREE: REIMBURSEMENT

Basic Insurance Principles

Health insurance companies act as the financial "middleman" between patients and medical providers. The consumer pays the insurance company a **premium**—a regular, predetermined amount of money. In return, the insurer covers some amount of the financial costs of the consumer's medical care. The types of services covered and the amount the insurance company will pay is determined by each person's individual health insurance plan.

Every customer that pays premiums to the insurance company is a risk and has the potential to cost the company money in the form of payouts for medical services. The premiums collected from multiple consumers are expected to offset these payout amounts and allow the insurance company to earn a profit. The insurance company may also earn investment returns on the premiums collected.

> Insurance companies hire case managers to help minimize the risk of making large payouts for individual customers. These case managers work with customers and medical providers to proactively avoid hospitalizations and other expensive care. They ensure that patients adhere to treatment plans, receive preventative care, and know the details of their health insurance plan.

Federal health insurance programs are available to some individuals, including people with disabilities or low incomes, veterans, and people over sixty-five. These programs do not require a premium, or require only a small premium, and are largely funded through taxes. The services covered under these programs are defined by federal and state laws and regulations.

PRACTICE QUESTION

1. John is diagnosed with congestive heart failure and is prescribed furosemide 20 mg by mouth twice daily. John goes to the local pharmacy and picks up his medicine at no cost. The cost of the medication is an example of what type of insurance payment?

    A) co-insurance

    B) deductible

    C) co-pay

    D) extra-contractual benefit

Managed Care Organizations

The majority of health care in the United States is provided through **managed care organizations (MCOs)**, which seek to control quality and costs by managing patients' use of medical services. MCOs use a variety of techniques to meet these goals. They contract with providers so their members can access their services at a discounted rate, and they may require patients to use only specific providers. MCOs may also require referrals or pre-approval for specialized medical care while easing access to lower-cost preventative care. They may also limit the amount paid for specific services or deny payment for services they feel are not medically necessary.

MCOs also minimize the money they pay out for a patient's medical care by sharing the cost of care with the patient.

In addition to the cost of their premium, patients share the cost of their medical expenses through payments that are referred to as co-pays, deductibles, and co-insurance. Co-pays are set payments that patients pay every time they seek medical care. For example, their insurance requires them to pay a $15 co-pay every time they see their medical provider.

A deductible is a set amount that patients must pay before the insurance company will cover any of their medical care. Typically, deductibles are much higher than co-pays, but the patient only has to pay it once a year. A patient could also have both a co-pay and a deductible. In that instance, if a patient has a deductible of $1,000 a year and a $250 co-pay for emergency room care, she will have to pay $1,000 of her emergency room care even if it only costs $1,001. If she needs additional emergency room care at any time during the remainder of the covered year, she would only have to pay the $250 co-pay no matter the total cost of the additional emergency room care.

Another way insurance companies share the cost of medical care with the patient is through co-insurance. Co-insurance is the total percentage an insurance company will pay for your medical care. If a patient has an insurance policy that has an 80 percent co-insurance, that means the insurance company will only pay 80 percent of the cost of the care regardless of the total amount. This is not a set amount; the amount the patient ends up paying depends on the total cost of care.

It is possible for a patient to have a co-insurance, a deductible, and a co-pay in one insurance policy. Fortunately, insurance policies usually come with a maximum out-of-pocket limit. An example of this would be a patient who has a maximum out-of-pocket limit of $5,000 per year, an 80/20 co-insurance, and a deducible of $1,500 for hospital care. If the patient experiences a costly medical problem and is admitted to the hospital, he will have to pay the $1,500 deductible and 20 percent of the cost of his care until he has paid an additional $3,500. If his care costs more than that or he ends up back in the hospital, the insurance company is responsible for paying for the rest.

There are four main types of MCOs available to patients:

+ preferred provider organization (PPO)
+ exclusive provider organizations (EPO)

- ✦ health maintenance organization (HMO)
- ✦ point-of-service (POS) plans

These plans exist on a spectrum that balances flexibility and cost. PPO health care plans offer the most flexibility but are also the most expensive. HMO plans offer the least flexibility but generally will be cheaper for the consumer.

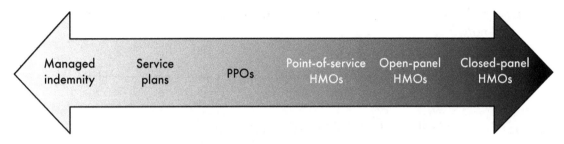

Figure 3.1. Spectrum of Managed Care

Preferred Provider Organizations

In a **preferred provider organization (PPO)**, providers contract with the insurance company to create a **network**. If the plan member sees medical professionals included in this network, the member receives the PPO's negotiated rate, which is usually substantially lower than the provider's cash rate. The insurer will then cover some portion of the cost (depending on the plan), and the member pays the specified co-insurance.

In a PPO, pre-authorization for medically necessary services may be required. In addition, the insurance company may not pay for a service that a physician requests if the company does not feel the service is medically necessary. For example, a PPO plan may not authorize payment for an expensive brand name prescription if a cheaper generic version is available.

 In a PPO, providers are usually compensated using a fee-for-service arrangement in which providers bill the insurance company for each separate service provided.

PPO plans allow plan members to go directly to a specialist without a referral from a primary care physician. However, prior authorization from the insurance company may be needed to ensure insurance coverage.

Members in a PPO may use the services of health care providers outside the network but will have to pay higher rates and will have a higher co-insurance and max out-of-pocket amount (which may not be limited for out-of-network services).

PPO plans typically have higher premiums than other health plans. Once members have met their annual deductible, the insurance company will pay a larger portion of the cost. If members meet their out-of-pocket maximum, the insurer will cover all approved health care costs. Deductibles and max out-of-pocket costs are usually lower for in-network care and much higher for out-of-network care.

PRACTICE QUESTION

2.   Mike recently signed up for a new PPO plan. He has an appointment with his primary care physician (PCP) and receives a call from the office informing him that the physician is not in Mike's network. Which of the following is true?

   A)   Mike can negotiate with his PCP to lower his out-of-pocket costs.

   B)   Mike will pay the same amount to see his PCP even though he is now out of network.

   C)   Mike can no longer see his PCP.

   D)   Mike cannot find a new PCP in-network since he already has a PCP.

EXCLUSIVE PROVIDER ORGANIZATIONS

An **exclusive provider organization (EPO)** also contracts with providers to form a network. The EPO will cover in-network health care services in the same manner as a PPO. However, out-of-network services are not covered except in cases of medical emergencies (once the patient is stable, the insurance plan may request to transfer to an alternative hospital within the network). Because the customer is responsible for all out-of-network costs, the premiums for an EPO plan are usually lower than those for a PPO.

A PCP referral is not needed for specialist services, but the customer is responsible for ensuring that all providers are in-network. Pre-authorization is usually required to have services approved for reimbursement.

PRACTICE QUESTION

3.   A client with chronic shoulder pain thinks he needs an MRI to identify the source of the pain. If the client has an EPO plan, who should the case manager suggest he contact to get pre-authorization for the MRI?

   A)   the insurance company

   B)   the client's primary care physician

   C)   an orthopedic specialist

   D)   a private MRI imaging center

HEALTH MAINTENANCE ORGANIZATIONS

A **health maintenance organization (HMO)** requires the member have a primary care physician who coordinates all care. Members may choose their own primary care physician from a list of in-network providers. However, if none are chosen, the insurance company will assign the member a PCP.

Referrals from the PCP are needed for any type of medical service, including specialist visits, diagnostic tests, and medical equipment. The primary care provider in an HMO contract is often referred to as a **gatekeeper**. They oversee all primary and preventative care. The gatekeeper authorizes referrals, lab studies, diagnostic testing, and hospitalization.

All medical providers also need to be in-network for the insurance company to pay for their services. If the gatekeeper refers the patient to a specialist and the patient attempts to see an alternative specialist, services will not be covered. Because HMOs can control costs by excluding out-of-network providers, their premiums are lower than those for a PPO or an EPO.

Providers are reimbursed by the HMO through an arrangement called **capitation**, in which providers are payed a fixed amount per member, per month. If a patient sees his HMO primary care physician several times in one month, the primary care physician is only paid the payment provided in the contract.

HMOs may have some services, called **carve-outs**, that are excluded from the capitation rate and are usually handled by a designated provider. Common carve-outs include mental health and addiction services, cancer treatments, and ambulance services. The insurance company's payment and pre-authorization policies may be different for carve-outs than for other covered specialist services.

There are four types of HMOs:

+ **staff model**: Physicians and other medical providers are direct employees of the HMO and only see patients who are members of that HMO.

+ **group model**: HMO contracts with multidisciplinary group practices that employ physicians and other medical providers. Providers may be limited to members of the HMO or may take outside patients.

+ **independent practice association model**: HMO contracts with independent practice associations to provide services.

+ **network model**: HMO contracts with a mix of private physicians, group practices, and independent practice associations.

PRACTICE QUESTION

4.   Capitation is a payment method in which
    A)   physicians are paid directly by the HMO.
    B)   services are bundled into a single payment.
    C)   out-of-network services are denied.
    D)   providers are paid a flat rate for each HMO member.

POINT-OF-SERVICE PLANS

Point-of-service (POS) health plans combine characteristics of HMO and PPO plans. As in an HMO plan, the member must designate a primary care physician to act as gatekeeper for medical services. The insurer will cover authorized, in-network services much like an HMO. However, the patient may choose to go out of network and pay higher out-of-pocket expenses. Typically, a POS plan will have a high deductible and co-insurance to encourage members to use in-network services. This type of health plan is designed for individuals who want the lower premiums and PCP-centered care of an HMO but also want some coverage for out-of-network costs.

5. Allison has a rare inflammatory disease and has had her care successfully managed by her PCP for many years. However, she would like to see an out-of-network rheumatologist who her PCP thinks may be able to help with her pain. What type of insurance plan would best suit her needs?

    A) HMO
    B) PPO
    C) EPO
    D) POS

Indemnity Insurance

Indemnity insurance does not use a network and instead allows members to use the services of any medical provider, including specialists. Indemnity plans provide a flat fee for services based on the **usual, customary, and reasonable rate (UCR)** for a specific location (and thus are sometimes called fee-for-service plans). For example, if an indemnity plan includes $5,000 in coverage for hospitalization costs, the plan will pay up to $5,000 for hospitalization at any location. However, the patient will be responsible for any additional costs. The patient may also be asked to pay medical costs up front and then be reimbursed by the insurer. In addition, most indemnity plans will include a deductible.

Indemnity plans used to be the main type of health insurance available but today are very rarely used as primary insurance. Instead, these policies are used as a supplemental policy to help cover co-pays, deductibles, and co-insurance fees accumulated from a primary managed care insurance plan. Some plans will cover only hospital-surgical costs, and others may cover other medical services.

 Some types of indemnity insurance can be used to cover non-medical expenses or make up for missed income due to illness or injury.

PRACTICE QUESTION

6. Which of the following statements from a client suggests that he may benefit from a secondary indemnity policy?

    A) I live in a rural region with a very small number of medical providers.
    B) I cannot afford high premiums or out-of-pocket expenses.
    C) I would like to keep my current PCP.
    D) I'm not sure how insurance works and am not very good at filling out paperwork.

Private Benefit Programs

Customers can purchase insurance plans through their employer as part of a group plan or through the health insurance marketplace established under the Affordable Care Act (ACA).

EMPLOYER-SPONSORED HEALTH COVERAGE

Companies may choose to offer health coverage through **employer-sponsored health coverage**. These plans are also called **group plans** because the same insurance coverage is offered to all members of the group (in this case, the employees). The employer picks the insurance policy and pays for part of the premiums. All employees within the business, and their dependents, are offered the insurance.

Employer-sponsored plans tend to have more comprehensive coverage and cost less than individually purchased plans. As a group, businesses can negotiate better rates for their members, and businesses will often offer high-quality benefit plans to recruit and retain employees.

The **Consolidated Omnibus Budget Reconciliation Act of 1985 (COBRA)** requires employers with twenty or more employees to offer employees and their dependents continued coverage if they have a qualifying event. These events include:

+ employee is laid off
+ divorce that ends spouse's eligibility for benefits
+ death of the employee
+ dependent child reaches the age at which benefits end

COBRA coverage is offered for up to 18 months. During this time, the insured person must pay the entire premium as well as an administration fee (usually 2 percent). This added expense can make COBRA coverage unaffordable for many people. Some states have passed legislation that extends COBRA coverage by applying regulations to smaller businesses or adding qualifying events.

PRACTICE QUESTION

7. An employee at a large company was recently laid off. Which of the following would be a good reason for her to enroll in COBRA coverage instead of an individual plan?

    A) Shopping for new health insurance is time consuming.

    B) She has already met her deductible for the year.

    C) She would like to save money.

    D) She needs to include dependents on her health insurance.

INDIVIDUALLY PURCHASED INSURANCE

Consumers can purchase individual health care plans through the **health care marketplace** (also called **health exchanges**). The **Patient Protection and Affordable Care Act (ACA)**, colloquially referred to as "Obamacare," regulates the type of insurance available through the marketplace. All plans available to consumers must meet the following requirements:

+ Plans must cover **essential health benefits**: ambulatory care, emergency services, hospitalization, maternity and newborn care, mental health and substance abuse services, prescription drugs, rehabilitative and habilitative services, laboratory services, preventive and wellness services, and pediatric services.

+ Plans cannot include an annual spending cap on essential health benefits spending.

+ No insurer may exclude customers or vary rates based on a customer's pre-existing conditions.

Individually purchased plans are managed care plans with the same structure as employer-based plans. They can be PPOs, HMOs, EMOs, or POS plans and can carry highly variable premiums, deductibles, co-insurance, and max out-of-pocket amounts. Plans are categorized as bronze, silver, gold, or platinum based on the level of insurance provided.

 Government subsidies for purchasing health care plans on the marketplace are available to individuals and families with low incomes.

Health care exchanges have an **open enrollment period** (typically from Nov. 1 to Dec. 15) during which individuals can purchase insurance. Customers can also purchase insurance from the exchange if they have a qualifying event (e.g., losing employer coverage).

PRACTICE QUESTION

8. A self-employed individual purchases a PPO plan through the health exchange. Which of the following services would the plan have to cover?

    A) chiropractic appointments for muscle pain

    B) hearing aids for congenital hearing loss

    C) dental exams and X-rays

    D) annual physicals

Public Benefit Programs

MEDICARE

The US federal government provides insurance for certain individuals through the **Medicare** program, which is administered through the Centers for Medicare and Medicaid Services (CMS). People eligible for Medicare include those who:

+ are sixty-five years or older and have paid payroll taxes

+ are younger than sixty-five and have a disability

+ have end-stage renal failure

+ have amyotrophic lateral sclerosis (ALS)

Medicare includes four parts. **Medicare Part A (hospital/hospice)** covers inpatient services, including hospitalization, rehabilitation or nursing services at a skilled nursing facility, and hospice care. Hospitalization is covered for up to ninety days, with co-insurance required after sixty days. Stays at a skilled nursing facility are covered for one hundred days with co-pays required after twenty days. Patients will only be covered after hospitalization and must receive medically necessary care or therapy; inpatient services solely for activities of daily living are not covered. Hospice services will be covered for patients with less than six months to live.

Medicare Part B (medical) covers outpatient services, including preventative services, diagnostic tests, outpatient procedures, emergency care treatment, home nursing and therapy visits, and some ambulance services. Part B also covers **durable medical equipment (DME)**, which is equipment that provides medical benefit to patients in their day-to-day life. DME must:

+ have a primarily medical purpose
+ be prescribed by a physician
+ be used at home
+ be for repeated use (durable)

Medicare Part C (Medicare Advantage plans) is administered through a private insurer that contracts with the government. These plans must include coverage for all services covered in both Medicare Part A and B. They are usually HMO-style plans with a network and PCP who acts as a gatekeeper; however, a small number are PPOs.

 Medicare Parts A – D have financial enrollment penalties if a person does not sign up when coverage first becomes available or if insurance coverage lapses.

Medicare Part D (prescription drug plans) is administered by private insurers or pharmacy benefits managers who provide prescription drug coverage. The insurer may choose which drugs to cover, but the CMS requires that insurers cover drugs from specific classes. In addition, the CMS also provides a list of drugs that it does not allow Part D plans to cover. Part D plans can be stand-alone prescription drug plans (PDPs) or can be bundled with Medicare Advantage (Part C) plans.

Medicare has a system of premiums, deductibles, and co-insurance that is similar to private insurance plans. These costs vary by part.

+ Medicare Part A has no premiums if the person or their spouse has paid Medicare taxes for ten years (forty quarters). People over sixty-five who do not meet the tax requirement may buy into Medicare by paying premiums. It also has a standard deductible and co-insurance amount set by the CMS.
+ Medicare Part B requires a monthly premium that is based on income. It also has a standard deductible set by the CMS. After meeting the deductible, patients will usually pay 20 percent of the cost of treatment (as set by Medicare).
+ The premiums, deductibles, and co-insurance for Medicare Parts C and D are set by the individual insurance plan purchased.
+ Neither Medicare Part A or B has an annual maximum out-of-pocket amount. Purchased plans for Parts C and D may set a maximum out of pocket.

9.   Mrs. Turner is about to turn sixty-five and is looking at Medicare plans. Twice a week she receives dialysis at the only clinic available in her small town. Which plan should she purchase to cover these treatments?

   A)   Medicare Part A

   B)   Medicare Part B

   C)   Medicare Part C

   D)   Medicare Part D

MEDICAID

Medicaid is a joint federal-state program that provides health coverage for individuals with low incomes. Because Medicaid is partially funded and regulated by states, eligibility and coverage vary widely by state. Generally, Medicaid will cover individuals with low incomes and has special provisions for coverage of pregnant people, children, the elderly, and people with disabilities.

 Medicaid also provides nursing home coverage that is not covered by Medicare.

The ACA expanded Medicaid coverage in 2014 to cover all individuals making 133 percent of the poverty line. However, the Supreme Court ruled that states could refuse to participate in the expansion, creating a division in Medicaid coverage between states that chose to expand and those that did not. In addition, some states have implemented cost-sharing measures such as premiums, co-insurance, and deductibles (these costs cannot be imposed for pregnancy-related services, emergency care, or preventative care for children).

Depending on state requirements, some people may qualify for both Medicare and Medicaid. For those with **dual eligibility**, Medicare must be billed first, with Medicaid billed secondary for services Medicare does not cover.

PRACTICE QUESTION

10.   Which of the following people is most likely to have dual eligibility for Medicare and Medicaid?

   A)   A twenty-five-year-old woman who has recently given birth to a child with a congenital heart disorder.

   B)   A twenty-year-old woman with end-stage renal disease who cannot purchase health insurance.

   C)   A sixteen-year-old boy who is addicted to opioids.

   D)   A retired sixty-five-year-old man who frequently travels out of the country.

SOCIAL SECURITY DISABILITY INSURANCE

Social Security Disability Insurance (SSDI) is a benefit program for people who are blind or disabled and cannot work. It is paid for out of the federal disability trust fund. To be eligible, you must have been employed for at least ten years or be the dependent of someone who has been employed for at least ten years. You must also be blind or fit the Social Security Administration's definition of permanently disabled. The amount SSDI recipients are paid depends solely on what they earned during their working years. If they are a dependent, the amount is based on their provider's earnings. After two years of being on SSDI, a patient is also eligible to receive federal health insurance through Medicare.

PRACTICE QUESTION

11. Which of the following people is most likely to be receiving SSDI benefits?

    A) a single mother raising a child with disabilities

    B) a nineteen-year-old construction worker recently diagnosed with a serious mental impairment

    C) an injured factory worker who is expected to return to an alternate job within nine months

    D) an administrative assistant with disabilities that affect her mobility

SUPPLEMENTAL SECURITY INCOME

Unlike SSDI, **Supplemental Security Income (SSI)** is a cash benefit for those who are disabled and have a limited income. It is paid for through tax revenues. Eligibility does not have any requirements regarding former employment. A recipient must meet the federal government's definition of *disabled* or *blind* or be older than sixty-five and have a limited income. Typically, because of their limited income, SSI beneficiaries are also immediately eligible for their state's Medicaid health insurance program.

PRACTICE QUESTION

12. A CCM has a client with disabilities. She should advise her client to apply for SSI if the client needs

    A) supplemental health insurance to cover physical therapy.

    B) additional income to supplement her earnings from a full-time job.

    C) additional income because her disability prevents her from working full time.

    D) supplemental health insurance to cover prescription medications.

Military Benefit Programs
TRICARE

TRICARE is a health care program for military personnel, including active duty US armed forces, those in the National Guard or military reserve, and military family members. Dependents and surviving spouses are also covered if the veteran was killed in active duty. The Department of Defense Health Agency manages the program, but health benefits are provided by a civilian provider network.

> 🔍 TRICARE was formerly known as CHAMPUS (Civilian Health and Medical Program of the Uniformed Services). In 1997, CHAMPUS become TRICARE (a managed care plan) to help cut costs and streamline administration.

TRICARE offers many different options. Costs vary and are based on the plan selected, whether the service member enlisted before or after January 1, 2018, and whether the member is currently on active duty, retired, or medically retired. Survivors are also eligible to enroll and pay the same rates as medically retired members. Premiums for TRICARE are referred to as enrollment fees and can be a one-time fee or a monthly fee, depending on the plan. Active duty members typically don't pay an enrollment fee. Deductibles, premiums, and max out-of-pocket rates are nothing for active duty TRICARE Prime members, but TRICARE For Life medically retired members pay a $300 premium, a $3,500 deductible, and a co-insurance of 20 percent for all in-network care and 25 percent for all out-of-network care with no cap.

+ **TRICACRE Prime** is a managed care plan and the least expensive plan available. It is for active duty members who live within Prime service areas in the US. Eligible enrollees include active duty military and their families, retired military and their families, Guard reserve members who have been on active duty for more than 31 consecutive days, non-activated Guard/reserve members and their families who qualify for Transitional Assistance benefits, retired Guard/reserve members age sixty and older and their families, surviving family members, Medal of Honor awardees and their families, and qualified ex-spouses of non-active military members and their families who live and receive their medical care within the US.

+ **TRICARE Prime Remote, TRICARE Prime Overseas**, and **TRICARE Prime Remote Overseas** are all managed care policies for active duty service members, including National Guard/reserve members who are ordered to active duty service for 31 or more consecutive days and family members who live with enrolled service members. Plan eligibility depends on where the member lives in relation to a military health care facility. **TRICARE Select** is a fee-for-service plan. The same members who are eligible for a Prime plan and receive their medical care within the US are eligible for the Select plan.

+ **TRICARE Select Overseas** is a fee-for-service plan that has more options but is more expensive than the Prime Overseas plans. The same members are eligible as above.

+ **TRICARE For Life** is accepted worldwide but a beneficiary must have Medicare A and B to be eligible. It is the secondary insurance for those on Medicare but acts as the primary insurance when Medicare is not accepted. It has no annual premium. There is a deductible of $150 for an individual and no more than $300 for a family for members who are medically retired or a surviving family member.

+ **TRICARE Reserve Select** is a managed care plan for reserve members that may be used with any TRICARE authorized provider, but services may require preauthorization.

+ **TRICARE Retired Reserve** is a PPO plan for qualified retired reserve members and surviving family members.

+ **TRICARE Young Adult** plans are open to eligible adult children of service members between the ages of twenty-one and twenty-six. Prime, Prime Overseas, and Prime Remote managed care options are available for the young adult policies as well as a Select PPO option similar to the general TRICARE policies with the same names.

+ **US Family Health Plan (USFHP)** and **TRICARE Young Adult** are managed care plans that require the service member to choose a provider for care, but the member cannot receive care from providers who are eligible for reimbursement through TRICARE, Medicare, or are a military medical provider.

TRICARE also offers other benefits, such as pharmacy and dental programs.

PRACTICE QUESTION

13. Which of the following people would NOT be eligible for TRICARE?

A) the widow of a uniformed service member who has remarried

B) the child of a uniformed service member who just turned twenty-one

C) a member of the National Guard

D) the six-year-old child of an Army serviceman

VETERANS HEALTH ADMINISTRATION

Once military service members retire or otherwise separate themselves from military service, the Veterans Health Administration will provide them and their dependents medical care at Veterans Administration (VA) medical facilities all over the US. Veterans are automatically eligible for services if they received an honorable discharge and served a minimum of 24 months in active duty or, for reserve members, the full length of their call-up to active duty during wartime. The minimum service requirement can be waived depending on the reason for discharge. Care is free for veterans who meet certain military service conditions or income guidelines. Veterans who make more than the income limit will be required to pay a co-pay.

Veterans who received a less than honorable discharge can apply for a discharge upgrade or a VA character review in order to get benefits. These can sometimes take up to a year to process. Veterans with a less than honorable discharge that are suffering from trauma or another mental illness related to their service, including sexual trauma, are immediately eligible for benefits regardless of their discharge status.

Health care provided by the VA includes primary and specialty care services, including mental health services, prescription coverage, surgeries, emergency room, and inpatient hospital care. Under certain conditions, the VA will also cover vision and dental care. The VA also provides reimbursement for travel to a VA medical center, covers home health or long-term care, and offers support services for caregivers.

In order to apply for VA health benefits, a veteran can submit the required forms online, in person, over the phone, or by mail. An eligibility letter should arrive in the mail one week after submission of the application. A short time later the veteran will receive a "welcome phone call" during which her benefits will be reviewed and her first appointment with a medical provider will be scheduled.

PRACTICE QUESTION

14. Which of the following people is MOST likely to be eligible for VA benefits?
     A) a person currently serving in the armed forces
     B) a veteran given a dishonorable discharge for desertion
     C) an army serviceman who has been discharged from active duty following an injury
     D) a retired mental health provider

CHAMPVA

CHAMPVA (the Civilian Health and Medical Program of the Department of Veterans Affairs) is another military health coverage benefit. CHAMPVA provides comprehensive health coverage for a spouse or dependent of a veteran who is permanently disabled due to military service, or a spouse or dependent of a veteran who was totally and permanently disabled due to a service-related injury at the time of death. The family members are also eligible for CHAMPVA if the military member died in the line of duty and the death was not caused by misconduct. Typically, those beneficiaries are eligible for TRICARE rather than CHAMPVA.

PRACTICE QUESTION

15. A veteran is 100 percent disabled due to a war event. Which type of health care coverage is he most likely to receive?
     A) TRICARE
     B) CHAMPVA
     C) Veterans Health Administration
     D) SSI

Pharmacy Benefits Management

A **pharmacy benefits manager** (PBM) is a third-party administrator that handles prescription medication claims for insurance companies and federal benefits programs. The goal of pharmacy benefit management is to reduce the amount customers and insurers spend on prescription medications. PBMs accomplish this goal through a variety of techniques:

  ✦ processing prescription claims
  ✦ maintaining a network of participating pharmacies

- ✦ negotiating drug costs
- ✦ managing patients' access to specialty medications
- ✦ obtaining rebates from drug manufacturers
- ✦ operating mail order pharmacies

Another major PBM duty is maintaining the **formulary**, a list of medications that are approved for reimbursement. Most formularies use a **tiered system** designed to encourage physicians and customers to choose lower-cost drugs. Tier 1 drugs are usually generic and available to the customer at little to no cost. Higher tier drugs are specialty or brand-name medications; the customer usually pays an escalating co-pay or co-insurance for drugs in each tier. Medications not on the formulary are not covered by the insurance or benefits providers, meaning the customer must pay the full price out of pocket.

 The three largest PBMs—Express Scripts, CVS Health (Caremark), and OptumRx (United Health)—handle 70 percent of all prescriptions filled in the US.

PRACTICE QUESTION

16. Which of the following prescriptions likely cost the customer the least amount of money out of pocket?

A) a thirty-day supply of a brand name medication picked up at the local pharmacy

B) a thirty-day supply of a tier 3 medication delivered by mail

C) a ninety-day supply of a tier 2 medication picked up at the local pharmacy

D) a ninety-day supply of a tier 1 medication delivered by mail

Workman's Compensation

Workman's compensation (also known as *workers' compensation*) is an insurance benefit that most employers are required to carry in most of the US. The only exception is the state of Texas. States determine which businesses must carry workman's compensation and the type of insurance carrier that can carry it. Workman's compensation provides medical benefits and a replacement income while an employee recovers from a work-related injury. If the injury results in a permanent disability, workman's compensation benefits would provide the employee with an income for a predetermined length of time or a lump sum compensation payment, medical benefits, and job retraining. If an employee is killed on the job, some states require a predetermined minimum benefit to be paid to the employee's dependents.

OSHA has defined a "work-related" injury as an injury occurring while the employee was performing a work-related task. When an employee is injured on the job, the employer is required to mail or give the employee a claim form and directions on how to file a workman's compensation claim within one business day of the injury being reported. Once the employee files the claim, the insurance company will then instruct the employee to see a medical doctor who will evaluate their injury. This MD then reports back to the insurance company on the severity of the injury and if the injury is work related. If it is determined that the employee's injury qualifies for workman's compensation, the employee can choose to claim these benefits. However, by claiming workman's compensation benefits, employees give up their right to sue their employer for any negligence regarding their injury.

PRACTICE QUESTION

17. Sarah has suffered an occupational injury and wishes to utilize her workman's compensation benefit. She is unable to speak due to her injury and needs family support. Who is most likely to file the First Report of Injury on Sarah's behalf?

   A) her family

   B) her employer

   C) her insurance carrier

   D) state regulators

Financial Resources

Medical care can be quite costly for many Americans. After an illness or injury, clients may be confronted by the double burden of large medical bills and lost income. The CCM should be prepared to help these clients access resources to meet their financial needs. A brief overview of available financial resources is listed below.

+ waiver program: a program provided by the Centers for Medicare and Medicaid Services that allows aged and disabled adults and children to remain in their home or a community setting and receive nursing home level of care

+ special needs trust: a trust for a disabled person that won't prevent that person from receiving Medicaid or SSI benefits

> Around 6 percent of people declaring bankruptcy in the United States do so directly because of medical bills. Many more are forced to declare bankruptcy because of loss of income following injury or illness.

+ viatical settlement: sale of a life insurance policy by the owner to a third party in order to receive a lump sum greater than the cash surrender amount but less than the net death amount

+ accelerated death benefit: a life insurance benefit that is paid if the policy holder is diagnosed with a terminal illness or an illness that greatly reduces the policy holder's lifespan

+ reverse mortgage: a loan for homeowners sixty-two years or older that uses the home equity for collateral and doesn't need to be repaid until the last surviving homeowner passes away or permanently moves out of the home

18. Alan is a sixty-five-year-old retiree whose granddaughter has multiple sclerosis. He would like to contribute to the cost of her medical care but does not want to prevent her from receiving SSI benefits. Which financial resource should Alan use?

A) special needs trust

B) viatical settlement

C) accelerated death benefit

D) reverse mortgage

Reimbursement and Payment Methodologies

With a **fee-for-service** reimbursement, each item involved in patient care is billed separately. If an insurance policy is not a managed care policy, it is typically a fee-for-service policy. Even a policy that uses a preferred provider organization (PPO) can be a fee-for-service policy. If, for example, a patient is to have a hip replacement, medical supplies, the hospital room, fees for surgeons and all other medical professionals involved, and anesthesia would be individually charged. By contrast, **bundled payments** are based on an episode of care that is reimbursed as one fee for all medical care provided. All items mentioned previously for the hip replacement surgery would be reimbursed in one lump sum.

Bundled payments for health care were created to encourage quality medical care and reduce health care costs. Many Medicaid insurances use bundled payments. The expected costs for all provider services are predetermined prior to the services being rendered. In order to make money, or at least not lose money, providers need to minimize complications and provide effective and efficient services to their patients. **Case rates** are a type of bundled payment. They are a flat fee typically paid by the day for a specific diagnosis, such as myocardial infarction. Bundled payments can also take the form of capitated payments. The payment made to the provider is based on a specific length of time and a specific number of patients. For example, an accountable care organization (ACO) may pay a primary care organization $3,500 per patient per month to manage all care for their patients.

Acute hospital patient satisfaction is monitored by the Centers for Medicare and Medicaid Services (CMS). Surveys used by CMS typically assess patient outcomes, aspects of a patient's experience, and efficiency of the hospital. Poor ratings in patient satisfaction can negatively impact a hospital's Medicare payments and brand reputation.

Medicare is a type of **prospective payment system**. The payments for patient services are determined according to the average cost of the services provided and the severity of the patient's diagnoses prior to treatment. The facility uses these predetermined rates to cover all services needed for a specific patient. The payment amounts for the same services will differ among patients depending on their diagnoses. If the care is inefficient or the patient suffers a preventable complication, like a hospital-acquired infection, or if the patient is readmitted to the hospital within a certain time frame, it will negatively impact the hospital's reimbursement for that patient. Hospitals that have multiple readmissions will be subject to decreased payments for all Medicare patients.

Medicare also utilizes a **value-based purchasing program** for acute care hospitals and physician services. The value-based purchasing program ensures Medicare beneficiaries receive quality medical care by rewarding well-performing hospitals with incentive payments for improved patient outcomes. The hospitals use a quality reporting program for specific measures, such as the mortality rate of patients with certain conditions, to determine the value of care provided by a specific facility. They also use a patient experience survey called the **Hospital Consumer Assessment of Healthcare Providers and Systems (HCAHPS)** to evaluate the value of the care patients are receiving and determine reimbursement and incentive rates for the facilities.

PRACTICE QUESTION

19. Which reimbursement method results in an itemized bill that lists the cost of each individual service provided during a medical procedure?

   A) prospective payment system

   B) episode of care

   C) fee for service

   D) case rate

Utilization Management

Controlling health care costs is a huge challenge, and many tools can assist with the process. **Utilization management** is focused on minimizing health care costs by using the most evidenced-based treatment that meets standards of care.

Utilization management is usually accomplished through utilization reviews. The first part of a utilization review verifies the patient's health plan coverage and determines if the service requested is a covered benefit. This is usually done through a verification of benefits by an employee of the medical facility or the service provider. If preauthorization is required for the service, the medical facility must submit the clinical evidence that the services are medically necessary to the insurance company, either verbally over the phone or by filling out an insurance form. Using the clinical evidence, the utilization reviewer will review the case and determine whether the clinical evidence meets medical necessity criteria for the services being sought. The case managers performing these insurance reviews are typically nurses educated on clinical care and medical terminology.

The provider that requests the service will be notified if medical necessity guidelines are met or not. If the service has been denied, the patient or provider may file an appeal. The appeals process may involve a first- and second-level appeal. If the patient is still denied coverage, the case may go to what is called a peer review. During a peer review, the patient's provider, a medical director, and an outside physician contracted with the insurance company will review the case again and make a final determination regarding approval.

A utilization review may be performed before medical care, over the course of medical care, or after completion of medical care. **Prospective review** is the process of ensuring medical necessity for a medical service before the service is performed. Prospective reviews are done when precertification is needed to ensure the patient is being treated at the appropriate level of care.

 The two most widely used products for utilization management guidelines are Milliman Care Guidelines and InterQual.

A **concurrent review** occurs when a patient's care continues to be monitored during medical care. The patient's care is compared to the expected course of treatment for their condition. Any additional services or service days needed while a patient is being treated must also be reviewed for medical necessity.

Retrospective review focuses on care after it has occurred. Clinical data is obtained and the service that has been received may be approved or denied by the insurance company. Using the clinical data, the patient's course of treatment is again assessed against the standards of care and the typical course of treatment for their procedure or illness. Retrospective review is important in the event of an emergency when precertification was not obtained.

PRACTICE QUESTION

20.   A patient has been admitted to the cardiac care unit (CCU) following a myocardial infarction. Which of the following medical providers would NOT play a role in the hospital's utilization management review for this patient?

A)   the attending physician in the CCU

B)   the patient's insurance provider

C)   the pharmacist who dispenses medications for the CCU

D)   the CCU's discharge planner

Models of Care

The US health care system continues to research and implement new **models of care** designed to improve the quality of care delivered to patients. These models often focus on integrating medical service providers into a single service that can help patients better manage their care and cut costs. Some of these models are discussed below. All of these models may use case managers to help coordinate care.

A **patient-centered medical home (PCMH)** is a health care delivery system based on centralized care coordination. The patient's personal physician oversees all of the patient's health care needs, including preventative care, inpatient care, and rehabilitation services. However, the personal physician does not act like an HMO gatekeeper: patients are free to see other providers within the service without a referral.

 Studies have shown that patients in a PCMH are up to 67 percent less likely to visit the ER than patients who use a standard model of care.

Accountable care organizations (ACOs) are groups of providers who together commit to meeting specific standards for quality of care. These standards address issues such as patient satisfaction, preventative health, and patient safety. Providers are financially incentivized to meet these standards, usually in the form of bonuses tied to cost savings (compared to a standard fee-for-service model). CMS initially developed ACOs for Medicare patients, but ACOs are now used by private insurers as well.

Medicaid patients with chronic health conditions may have their care coordinated by a **health home.** These networks of providers service Medicaid patients with

+ two chronic conditions

+ one chronic condition and high risk for a second

+ one serious and chronic mental health condition

Health homes focus on improving outcomes and cutting costs for these patients by coordinating care between all of the patient's medical providers, including PCPs, specialists, and social workers. Health homes are unique in that they also help patients access necessities such as transportation, housing assistance, and counseling.

Special needs plans (SNPs) are specialized Medicare Advantage plans that offer coordinated care to individuals who

+ are institutionalized

+ have dual eligibility

+ have specific chronic health conditions

These plans have benefits, networks, and formularies that are tailored to meet the needs of specific populations (e.g., patients in long-term care facilities or those with chronic heart failure).

The **chronic care model** addresses specific issues relevant to the care of individuals with multiple chronic conditions that create intensive health care needs. The model includes a framework to improve the following areas of care:

+ health systems (e.g., culture and organizational structure)

+ decision-making based on evidence and patient preference

+ clinical information systems to organize data

+ patient self-management support

+ patient access to community resources

+ delivery system for care, including care coordination

> CMS offers chronic care management (CCM) fees to providers who document at least twenty minutes of monthly non-face-to-face interaction with patients as part of a coordinated chronic care plan.

PRACTICE QUESTION

21. The primary factor that improves patient outcomes in a patient-centered medical home (PCMH) is

    A) coordination of care between providers.

    B) increased compensation for providers.

    C) access to new medications and procedures.

    D) providing patients with access to community resources.

Coding Methodologies

A universal set of codes is used to simplify health care communication, particularly for reimbursement. These medical codes alphanumerically define diagnoses, procedures, equipment, and services for health care professionals, insurance companies, and government health programs.

INTERNATIONAL CLASSIFICATION OF DISEASES

The **International Classification of Diseases (ICD)** is a coding system used to systematically classify diseases. It was created by the International Statistical Institute but was entrusted to the World Health Organization (WHO) in 1948. The most recent version currently in use is the ICD 10. Each ICD code corresponds to a different medical diagnosis. The codes are used to facilitate the identification and grouping of diseases for billing, disease monitoring, and other research or public health purposes. There are multiple coding reference books that have the complete list of ICD 10 codes on the market, but the ICD 10 reference book can also be ordered for free or accessed for free through a search application on the WHO website.

The ICD 10 codes are all alphanumeric. The first character is always a letter and the second character is always a number. The rest of the code could contain between one and five more characters, which could be a letter or a number, and there is always a decimal after the first three characters. For example, the ICD 10 code for fatty changes of the liver is K76.0, but nonalcoholic fatty liver inflammation is K75.81.

The ICD 11 is the most recent version of the ICD classification system. WHO released it in June 2018, but it will not go into effect until January 1, 2022.

Basic knowledge of the ICD coding system is important for medical case managers. Helping patients understand their medical bills is often a large part of meeting their care needs. The

CCM may collect data such as ICD codes, and apply this data to facilitate a smooth health care experience.

PRACTICE QUESTION

22. All of the following are important reasons for accurate coding using the ICD system EXCEPT

   A) tracking disease trends within and across communities.

   B) preventing the patient for being billed for the wrong diagnosis.

   C) ensuring the patient will receive care from the correct physician.

   D) improving hospital quality control.

CURRENT PROCEDURAL TERMINOLOGY

Current Procedural Terminology (CPT) uses a set of standardized five-digit codes to identify medical, surgical, or diagnostics services. CPT codes refer only to medical procedures and are used in conjunction with ICD codes (which gives the diagnosis for the underlying medical condition). The CPT coding system was developed by the American Medical Association (AMA), which releases updated codes every October.

 Case managers can be reimbursed using different CPT codes based on the services they provide, such as:

99495: transitional care management services of moderate complexity with a face-to-face visit within fourteen days of discharge.

99487: first hour of clinical staff time for chronic care management with no face-to-face time.

CPT is divided into three categories of codes:

  ✦ Category I is for common medical procedures that are widely used. This category includes the evaluation and management, surgical, medical, surgery, anesthesia, radiology, pathology, and laboratory codes.

  ✦ Category II codes are optional and are used for tracking and performance monitoring. For example, they document an assessment of tobacco use or blood pressure measurement.

  ✦ Category III codes are temporary codes for new procedures or technology that is involved in research.

Case managers do not usually do medical coding, but they need to be familiar with CPT/ICD codes and know how to read bills and reports containing these codes. For example, the CCM may need to review a client's bill to ensure he is being charged correctly. CCMs may also need to utilize CPT or ICD codes when doing quality control or utilization management in a hospital setting.

PRACTICE QUESTION

23. Which of the following does not have a CPT code?

A) venipuncture

B) MRI

C) myocardial infarction

D) CABG

DIAGNOSIS-RELATED GROUP

To simplify reimbursement and reduce costs, Medicare pays a predetermined amount for a given diagnosis while a patient is hospitalized, a system called the **inpatient prospective payment system (IPPS)**. The **diagnosis-related group (DRG)** is a classification system used to determine payments in the IPPS.

Medicare uses **Medicare Severity Diagnosis Related Groups (MS-DRGs)** to classify patients. The DRG is assigned to the patient based on

+ the primary diagnosis

+ secondary diagnoses

+ surgical procedures performed during the hospital stay

+ complications and comorbidities (CC) or major complications and comorbidities (MCC)

Each DRG is a three-digit number that describes a specific diagnosis (e.g., 176: pulmonary embolism without MCC). Medicare then determines the cost of the average resources used to treat patients in that DRG and pays the hospital a flat rate for each patient assigned that DRG. This process means that the hospital is paid the same amount for every patient hospitalized with the same DRG. Medicare's use of DRGs is designed to incentivize hospitals to provide only necessary care.

Other organizations have developed more complex DRG systems that incorporate factors such as the severity of the illness, the age and sex of the patient, and the patient's status at discharge. Some hospitals use these for billing outside the Medicare program. These systems include

+ All Patient DRGs (AP-DRGs)

+ All Patient Refined DRGs (APR-DRG)

+ International Refined DRGs (IR-DRG)

PRACTICE QUESTION

24. What characteristic would be considered when placing patients into a diagnostic-related group?

A) their income

B) their living environment

C) the reason they were admitted to the hospital

D) the number of children they have

Diagnostic and Statistical Manual of Mental Disorders

The **Diagnostic and Statistical Manual of Mental Disorders (DSM)** is published by the American Psychiatric Association. It is a manual that lists the symptoms of psychiatric disorders and their related states and provides guidelines regarding differential diagnosis of mental disorders and how to determine the severity of a diagnosis (e.g., length of time symptoms have been present, number of symptoms present). The DSM-5, published in 2013, is the most recent version. Clinicians and researchers use the DSM as a diagnostic tool. Like medical diagnoses, the diagnoses in the DSM have corresponding ICD 10 codes, so clinicians can use ICD 10 codes to bill for services.

PRACTICE QUESTION

25. Which of the following diagnoses can be found in the DSM-5?

A) reactive attachment disorder

B) myocardial infarction

C) irritable bowel syndrome

D) racing thoughts

Negotiation Techniques

While many costs and covered services are set in advance by managed care contracts, case managers may still be called on to negotiate the cost of medical care, length of stay, or covered services on behalf of clients, hospitals, or other employers. For example, the CCM may want a client's insurer to cover a bill for an out-of-network procedure through a single case agreement. To do this, the CCM will need to negotiate with the insurance company to find a compromise.

To be a successful negotiator, CCMs must be prepared. They need to be familiar with the patient's clinical data and the definition of medical necessity for the requested services. They also need to be familiar with certain laws regarding insurance coverage, such as the Mental Health Parity and Addiction Equity Act and the Affordable Care Act's ten essential benefits.

The CCM should begin negotiations with a cooperative attitude as opposed to an aggressive approach. They should be transparent and reasonable and strive to establish a relationship with the other parties. Active listening as well as clear communication is vital to a successful negotiation. Once areas of disagreement are discussed, the CCM should begin to work toward finding a common goal and focus on compromise. If this is not successful or the reviewer seems to be uncompromising, the CCM must remain civil; it is likely that they will encounter this insurance reviewer again. The CCM should always remember that there are many steps in the process, and no one conversation is the sole determinant of an outcome.

The CCM may also have to negotiate with the patient, the provider, or the patient's family members to develop a more realistic care plan. This may include suggesting more conservative treatment interventions or providing education on what conditions meet the insurance company's approval criteria for the level of care or services being sought. The CCM should be respectful of the patient's and provider's points of view while educating them about evidenced-based care and more realistic treatment interventions based on the best interests of the patient.

PRACTICE QUESTION

26. Alice was awarded a tier reduction for the price of a high-cost medication. She would like to be reimbursed for her out-of-pocket cost for the medication that she has paid for the entire year. The CCM can best help her by

A) calling the pharmacy and negotiating a lower cost for the medication.

B) calling the insurance company to determine what Alice needs to do to receive reimbursement.

C) calling the provider to report the complication and request medication samples.

D) contacting the medication's manufacturer to find available subsidies or coupons.

Answer Key

1. A) Incorrect. Co-insurance refers to the percentage amount paid by the insurance company after the deductible is met.

   B) Incorrect. The deductible is money that is paid by the insured before the insurance company pays.

   C) Correct. John has a zero-dollar co-pay for tier 1 medications such as furosemide.

   D) Incorrect. Extra-contractual benefits are benefits not covered by the insurance company.

2. **A) Correct.** Mike can attempt to negotiate with his PCP to see if he can pay a lower rate. Some doctors are willing to lower their cash rate to maintain continuity of care.

   B) Incorrect. Now that his PCP is out of network, Mike will have to pay a higher co-pay and will have a higher deductible for services.

   C) Incorrect. Mike can continue to see his PCP, but insurance will not cover as much of the cost.

   D) Incorrect. Within a PPO, patients may switch PCPs whenever they want.

3. A) Incorrect. The insurance company will require a physician to complete the pre-authorization paperwork.

   B) Incorrect. Depending on the situation, the PCP may be able to submit a pre-authorization form, but the insurance company will most likely ask for a specialist's assessment.

   C) Correct. An in-network orthopedic specialist will be able to assess the patient and submit a pre-authorization form that explains the need for the MRI. Because the client has an EPO, he can see the specialist without first seeing his PCP.

   D) Incorrect. Pre-authorization requires a physician and is not usually done by private diagnostic companies such as labs and imaging centers.

4. A) Incorrect. The process of capitation does not specify who is paid. For example, in a group model HMO, the HMO pays the group, which in turn pays physicians.

   B) Incorrect. Bundled payments are a separate type of payment arrangement from capitation.

   C) Incorrect. Capitation is not specific to in- or out-of-network payments.

   D) Correct. In a capitation arrangement, the HMO compensates providers with a flat fee for each member who uses their services.

5. A) Incorrect. With an HMO, her insurer would not cover any of the cost to see the specialist.

   B) Incorrect. Allison would like to keep her PCP to coordinate her care, so a PPO would not be the best choice for her.

C) Incorrect. As with an HMO, her insurer will likely not cover the cost of the specialist under an EPO plan.

D) **Correct.** With a POS plan, Allison can keep her PCP and pay lower premiums while still receiving some coverage to see a specialist.

6. A) **Correct.** Access to a very limited number of providers may be a reason to have an indemnity policy because the client can see any doctor available.

B) Incorrect. Indemnity policies typically have higher premiums and may require substantial out-of-pocket expenses.

C) Incorrect. The client will likely be able to keep his PCP with a PPO or POS plan, so he does not need a secondary indemnity plan.

D) Incorrect. Indemnity plans often require members to closely manage their health care expenses and reimbursements, so they would not be recommended for this client.

7. A) Incorrect. Although this statement is true, it is generally not a good reason to enroll in COBRA without exploring other options.

B) **Correct.** If the deductible has already been met, the employee may save money by staying on the same insurance plan.

C) Incorrect. The employee will likely find a marketplace plan that costs less than COBRA coverage.

D) Incorrect. The employee will be able to find plans for all family members through the marketplace, likely at a cheaper rate.

8. A) Incorrect. Chiropractors are not an essential health benefit and may not be covered.

B) Incorrect. Coverage for medical equipment and accommodations will vary by state and plan, so hearing aids may not be covered.

C) Incorrect. Adult dental coverage must be purchased separately through the health exchange.

D) **Correct.** Preventative care, including annual physicals, is included as an essential health benefit in plans purchased through a health exchange.

9. A) Incorrect. Medicare Part A covers inpatient services.

B) **Correct.** Medicare Part B covers outpatient services such as dialysis. Because Part B plans are optional and must be purchased, Mrs. Turner should plan to enroll in a Part B plan as soon as she is eligible.

C) Incorrect. Most Medicare Part C plans are HMOs, which may not cover the only clinic she has access to.

D) Incorrect. Medicare Part D plans cover prescription drugs.

10. A) Incorrect. The woman is not old enough to receive Medicare.

B) **Correct.** People with end-stage renal disease qualify for Medicare. She may also qualify for Medicaid because her income is low.

C) Incorrect. The teen may qualify for Medicaid due to his age but will not qualify for Medicare.

D) Incorrect. The man is old enough to qualify for Medicare. However, if he travels frequently, he likely does not meet the income requirement for Medicaid.

11. A) Incorrect. The mother is not disabled and cannot receive SSDI.

B) Correct. The teen is old enough to receive SSDI and may receive benefits if his mental impairment prevents him from working.

C) Incorrect. Workers who will return to work in less than a year are not eligible for SSDI.

D) Incorrect. People who are able to work are not eligible for SSDI.

12. A) Incorrect. SSI is a cash benefit, not health insurance.

B) Incorrect. She has full-time job and may not be eligible for SSI.

C) Correct. She has a limited income and may be eligible for SSI based on her disability.

D) Incorrect. SSI is a cash benefit, not health insurance.

13. **A) Correct.** Widows and surviving spouses who remarry are no longer eligible for TRICARE.

B) Incorrect. Children of uniformed service members may be eligible for TRICARE for Young Adults until age twenty-six.

C) Incorrect. Members of the National Guard are eligible for TRICARE.

D) Incorrect. Children of uniformed service members are eligible for TRICARE.

14. A) Incorrect. Active-duty personnel are not eligible for VA benefits.

B) Incorrect. Veterans who separated with a dishonorable discharge are not eligible for VA benefits.

C) Correct. Service members who have been honorably discharged are eligible for VA benefits.

D) Incorrect. VA benefits are only available to those who served on active duty in the US military.

15. **A) Correct.** This is a military health care coverage plan.

B) Incorrect. This is military coverage for spouses and dependents of a disabled veteran.

C) Incorrect. This is an integrated health care system.

D) Incorrect. This is a cash benefit.

16. A) Incorrect. Brand-name medications are more expensive than generics, and the patient did not save money by having the medication delivered by mail.

B) Incorrect. Tier 3 medications are the most expensive.

C) Incorrect. Tier 2 medications cost more than tier 1 medications and are usually more expensive when picked up at a pharmacy.

D) **Correct.** Tier 1 medications cost the least, and the customer likely saved money by having it delivered by mail.

17. A) Incorrect. It is not the responsibility of her family.

B) **Correct.** The employer is responsible.

C) Incorrect. The employer notifies the insurance carrier.

D) Incorrect. It is not the responsibility of the state regulators.

18. **A)** **Correct.** A special needs trust would allow Alan to set aside money for his granddaughter's medical care that would not prevent her from receiving SSI benefits.

B) Incorrect. Giving his granddaughter the profits from selling his life insurance policy would prevent her from accessing SSI benefits.

C) Incorrect. Alan does not have a terminal diagnosis, so he is not eligible for accelerated death benefits.

D) Incorrect. Alan is eligible for a reverse mortgage, but gifting the money to his granddaughter would prevent her from accessing SSI benefits.

19. A) Incorrect. A prospective payment system provides a predetermined reimbursement amount based on the average cost of the care needed for a specific service regardless of the intensity of care the patient ultimately needed.

B) Incorrect. An episode of care is a medical treatment event that includes all medical services needed for a specific medical condition.

C) **Correct.** Fee for service is a payment system that pays for each aspect of care separately.

D) Incorrect. Case rate is a type of bundled payment based on the type of patient and the typical care needed for a specific condition, such as a myocardial infarction.

20. **C)** **Correct.** Physicians, insurance companies, and discharge planners will all play a role in utilization management. The pharmacist will not.

21. **A)** **Correct.** PCMHs coordinate care to improve patients' health outcomes.

B) Incorrect. Increased compensation based on health outcomes is not generally part of a PCMH.

C) Incorrect. PCMHs focus on care coordination, not access to new medical services.

D) Incorrect. While some PCMHs may help patients access community resources, this is not the primary factor that improves patient outcomes.

22. A) Incorrect. The ICD system allows medical researchers to track trends in diseases and injuries.

B) Incorrect. In the US, medical billing relies on the ICD codes.

C) **Correct.** ICD codes are not used to verify whether a patient receives treatment from the correct physician.

D) Incorrect. ICD codes are used by hospital quality control personnel to track patient diagnoses.

23. A) Incorrect. Venipuncture (for a blood draw) is a diagnostic procedure with the CPT code 36415.

B) Incorrect. An MRI is a diagnostic test; it has different CPT codes depending on the type of MRI.

C) **Correct.** Myocardial infarction is a diagnosis and does not have a CPT code; it has an ICD code.

D) Incorrect. CABG (coronary artery bypass grafting) is a surgical procedure with various CPT codes for the type of CAGB performed.

24. A) Incorrect. A patient's income is a social determinant of health but is not considered in DRG placement.

B) Incorrect. A patient's living environment does impact illness, but it is not a consideration for a DRG placement.

C) **Correct.** The patient's diagnosis or scheduled procedure is a consideration for a DRG placement.

D) Incorrect. The number of children a patient has does not factor into a DRG.

25. A) **Correct.** Reactive attachment disorder is a trauma-related mental disorder.

B) Incorrect. Myocardial infarction is a medical diagnosis.

C) Incorrect. Irritable bowel syndrome is a medical diagnosis.

D) Incorrect. Racing thoughts are a symptom, not a diagnosis.

26. A) Incorrect. Alice has already received a cost reduction for the medication; trying to lower it further will not help Alice get reimbursed for previous prescriptions.

B) **Correct.** The CCM can use her expertise to communicate her client's need to the insurance company and complete the necessary paperwork.

C) Incorrect. The provider will likely not be able to help Alice get reimbursement from her insurance company.

D) Incorrect. While this may lower the out-of-pocket cost of medications, it will not help Alice get reimbursed.

FOUR: PSYCHOSOCIAL CONCEPTS AND SUPPORT SYSTEMS

Behavioral Change Theories and Stages

Some researchers, scientists, and behavior experts believe individuals drive behaviors. Others believe that it is the behaviors themselves that trigger or change other behaviors. The **transtheoretical model (TTM)** developed by researchers James Prochaska and Carlo DiClemente offers a useful perspective on the birth and growth of behavioral change. It defines a five-step process that is determined by an individual's readiness or willingness to change:

1. precontemplation stage (not ready to change)
2. contemplation stage (getting ready to change)
3. preparation stage (ready to change)
4. action stage (performing the action that will bring about change)
5. maintenance stage (integrating the action into one's lifestyle and making it habit)

> A case manager must assess readiness and willingness to change while managing all types of clients, as this step in the plan of care determines how successful the individual will be in self-managing his or her health condition(s).

PRACTICE QUESTION

1. Gene is a forty-eight-year-old male who someday wishes to stop smoking. He has given fleeting thought to it, but he still very much enjoys his two-pack-a-day habit and will not listen when his daughter lectures him about quitting. What stage of the transtheoretical model is Gene in now?

    A) contemplation stage

    B) precontemplation stage

    C) maintenance stage

    D) action stage

Interview Techniques

The purpose of a client interview is to collect relevant health information to determine the correct treatment plan. When a case manager (CCM) is preparing to interview a client, he or she must review the following in order to get the clearest possible picture of the client's health status:

+ client's health history
+ recent hospitalizations and emergency department visits
+ current medication list
+ alcohol or substance abuse history

The case manager must be engaging to develop a rapport with the client during the initial interview; this includes active listening and matching the client's communication style. Establishing a rapport with a client is important in making them feel more comfortable with the case manager. This will create a relationship in which the client is willing to share more information.

At the end of the interview, the case manager should summarize the gathered information and highlight important points for the client to ensure that nothing was missed. The CCM should also give the client the opportunity to ask questions. The case manager will then let the client know when to expect further contact. The CCM should provide direct contact information, should the client have any questions or concerns.

In behavioral health interviewing, the client may have a mental disability that prevents productive interviewing. A family member or guardian may assist in obtaining all pertinent information to establish a care plan. The care plan will be the foundation to develop a treatment strategy with achievable goals for the client.

PRACTICE QUESTION

2. Anna is a case manager who will contact a client for an initial interview. She should do all of the following EXCEPT

   A) review recent hospitalizations.

   B) examine client's provider information.

   C) enter a utilization review (UR) request for the client.

   D) review client's substance abuse history.

Assessment

HEALTH LITERACY ASSESSMENT

A **health literacy assessment** evaluates how well an individual can acquire, manage, and comprehend the fundamental health information and services required to make well-informed health decisions. The **Rapid Estimate of Adult Literacy in Medicine (REALM)** form uses word recognition to provide health care professionals with a reliable and quick estimation of a client's proficiency in health literacy. During the REALM exam, the interviewer gives the individual a list of random medical terms and asks him or her to read the terms aloud. The test taker can say "pass" if he or she does not know a word and proceed to the next word. Scoring is based on how many words the participant pronounces correctly.

Patient Name/ Subject # _____	Date of birth _____	Reading level _____
Date _____ Clinic _____ Examiner _____		Grade Completed _____
List One	**List Two**	**List Three**
fat	fatigue	allergic
flu	pelvic	menstrual
pill	jaundice	testicle
dose	infection	colitis
eye	exercise	emergency
stress	behavior	medication
smear	prescription	occupation
nerves	notify	sexually
germs	gallbladder	alcoholism
meals	calories	irritation
disease	depression	constipation
cancer	miscarriage	gonorrhea
caffeine	pregnancy	inflammatory
attack	arthritis	diabetes
kidney	nutrition	hepatitis
hormones	menopause	antibiotics
herpes	appendix	diagnosis
seizure	abnormal	potassium
bowel	syphilis	anemia
asthma	hemorrhoids	obesity
rectal	nausea	osteoporosis
incest	directed	impetigo
		Score
		List One _____
		List Two _____
		List Three _____
		Raw score _____

Figure 4.1. The Rapid Estimate of Adult Literacy in Medicine (REALM)

The **Test of Functional Health Literacy in Adults (TOFHLA)** measures reading comprehension and skill and was developed to evaluate adult literacy in a health care environment.

Table 4.1. Test of Functional Literacy in Adults (TOFHLA)

Description	Assesses literacy using materials related to health care
Time Length	Full version (TOFHLA): 18 – 22 minutes
	Short version (S-TOFHLA): 7 – 10 minutes
Scoring	0 – 53: inadequate health literacy
	54 – 66: marginal health literacy
	67 – 100: adequate health literacy

The first portion of the TOFHLA focuses on reading comprehension and is composed of a short paragraph that the client must read. At the completion of that task, the client is asked several questions relating to what he or she just read. This is used to determine if a client can grasp instructions about diagnostic procedures.

The skill (numeracy) portion of the assessment evaluates the client's understanding of such things as prescription labels and glucometer readings. Scoring is based on how well the individual answered the reading comprehension and prescription label questions.

 Health literacy assessment tools are important for a case manager to establish how well a client understands diagnostic procedures, discharge planning, and medication labels.

The **Newest Vital Sign Screening Tool (NVS)** is available in English and Spanish and consists of showing clients an ice cream nutrition label and asking six questions that pertain to the information on the label. Scoring is simple and is calculated by how many questions each client correctly answered, with one point being given for each correct answer. A score of 0 – 1 indicates low literacy, 2 – 3 is moderate literacy, and 4 – 6 is considered adequate literacy.

PRACTICE QUESTION

3. Katy is a case manager with a twenty-three-year-old Spanish-speaking client who has diabetes. She plans to work with her client on building new eating habits to help manage her condition. Which health literacy assessment tool should she use?

A) Rapid Estimate of Adult Literacy in Medicine (REALM)

B) Test of Functional Health Literacy in Adults (TOFHLA)

C) Short Test of Functional Health Literacy in Adults (S-TOFHLA)

D) The Newest Vital Sign (NVS)

PSYCHOLOGICAL AND NEUROPSYCHOLOGICAL ASSESSMENT

A **psychological assessment** is used to assess and treat psychological, psychiatric, and personality disorders, as well as developmental delays. A **neuropsychological assessment** can be used to measure capacity with regard to memory, reasoning, concentration, motor skills, and other cognitive elements. Psychological testing can be further categorized into four main types: clinical interview, assessment of intellectual functioning (IQ), personality assessment, and behavioral assessment.

The **clinical interview** is a basic but integral component of any psychological testing. Also known as an intake or admission interview, it is generally a comprehensive assessment to collect information about an individual's background and family relationships. Only a licensed psychologist may perform a clinical interview.

The **intellectual functioning (IQ test)** is used to measure typical intelligence and is further divided into subsections that evaluate verbal comprehension, perceptual reasoning, working memory, and processing speed.

The **personality assessment** was developed to help health care professionals gain better insight into an individual's personality. Two different types of objective tests used to evaluate this are the Minnesota Multiphasic Personality Inventory (MMPI-2) and the Sixteen Personality Factor Questionnaire (16PF).

The **Minnesota Multiphasic Personality Inventory (MMPI-2)** assesses personality traits such as paranoia, social introversion, and psychopathology, to name a few. It is not generally used to evaluate people with healthy personalities; rather, it measures dysfunction within an individual's personality.

The **Sixteen Personality Factor Questionnaire (16PF)** focuses on sixteen fundamental personality characteristics and functions to assist an individual in comprehending where their personality may register among those characteristics. The behavioral assessment serves to provide greater understanding of an individual's behavior and causative factors or thought processes behind those behaviors.

Certain instruments and assessments have been designed to measure psychological functioning. The **Rancho Los Amigos Level of Cognitive Functioning Scale (LCFS)** is a tool used to determine the level of brain function in post-comatose clients and clients with a closed head injury (including traumatic brain injury). It focuses on eight areas of cognition (awareness), with each level representing a progression of improvement from brain trauma or damage:

1. No response (score given of 1)
2. Generalized response (score given of 2)—reacts inconsistently with no purpose
3. Localized response (score given of 3)—reacts specifically to various stimuli, with different response each time
4. Confused-agitated response (score given of 4)—active but does not comprehend what has happened
5. Confused, inappropriate, non-agitated response (score given of 5)—less agitated, consistent reactions to basic commands
6. Confused-appropriate response (score given of 6)—motivated, highly dependent on others, more aware of self and loved ones
7. Automatic-appropriate response (score given of 7)—acts appropriately in the health care setting and at home; self-aware, oriented to place and time

8. Purposeful-appropriate response (score given of 8)—independently functions well within the world, has memory of how the past fits with the present and future

The **Mini-Cog assessment tool** is administered in three minutes to screen for cognitive deficiency in elderly adults within the principal health care environment and mainly concentrates on recall abilities. An individual is asked to remember three simple words, then is intentionally distracted by the examiner and later asked to repeat the three words given.

 The Mini-Cog instrument is widely used to assess memory recall in Alzheimer's clients.

PRACTICE QUESTION

4. Eleanor is a seventy-three-year-old female who recently fell in her bathroom and hit her head on the corner of her sink. She is currently comatose, and the Ranchos Los Amigos LCFS is being used to assess the level of impairment. When an ice cube is placed in her palm, she shivers. When it is placed in the same palm again, she flexes the hand holding the ice cube. This is an example of which type of response?

   A) localized response

   B) confused-appropriate response

   C) purposeful-appropriate response

   D) no response

Client Engagement and Self-Care Management

Client engagement is defined as connecting with a client in such a way that the client feels comfortable interacting with the CCM and is ready to take an active role in their own health care. When clients are truly engaged, they will begin to make changes to reach a goal of optimum health. **Client activation** is the knowledge and confidence that inspires clients to adequately and appropriately manage their health and make sound decisions related to health care. **Client empowerment** is defined as involving the client in the selection of the best health care management options by keeping the client well informed of all available choices while simultaneously considering their social situation and demands. Employing these practices while assisting a client in managing their care is instrumental in the client's compliance, positive progression toward care plan goal achievement, and outcome improvement. Ultimately, clients are "in the driver's seat" and directing all aspects of their care.

Self-care and **self-management** can be used interchangeably to refer to the desire, willingness, and capacity to care for oneself and manage one's health care. Case managers continually monitor their clients' abilities to care for themselves by evaluating lab results, changes in medications and dosages, and any changes in the clients' condition. A return demonstration of how to operate medical equipment or how to perform proper hygiene may also be needed.

Self-advocacy generally refers to supporting one's own needs and desires when they concern health care options. **Self-directed care** fits right in with self-advocacy, as it is care that is directed and therefore supported by the individual. **Informed decision-making** means ensuring that the client has all the information available to make an appropriate, well-informed medical decision. **Shared decision-making** involves collaboration between the client, the client's family or loved ones, and the managing physician to determine the best health care options for the client. These practices, used in conjunction with each other, help to promote the most optimal outcomes for the client, as he or she is always kept informed of new developments and never feels left out of the health care loop.

PRACTICE QUESTION

5. Sam is speaking with his case manager about his hypertension and mentions that he does not have a blood pressure monitor at home. What should the case manager do to help Sam self-advocate and manage his care?

   A) call Sam's family member and report that Sam needs a blood pressure monitor

   B) encourage Sam to call his primary care provider to ask for a prescription for a monitor

   C) provide Sam with a pamphlet on the importance of closely monitoring his blood pressure

   D) help Sam speak with his insurance provider about acquiring a blood pressure monitor

Psychosocial Elements of Case Management
BEHAVIORAL HEALTH CONCEPTS

The field of behavioral health is broad. A case manager who wants to successfully case manage individuals with behavioral health issues will need to understand the symptoms, treatments, and interventions for a range of behavioral and mental health disorders. Such disorders may include depression, anxiety, bipolar disorder, dissociative identity disorder, personality disorders, schizophrenia, attention deficit/hyperactivity disorder (ADHD), eating disorders, addictive disorders, and learning and conduct disorders.

The case manager caring for an individual with one or more behavioral health disorders must:

   1. complete a thorough health history and assessment (focusing on current behavioral health diagnoses and providers seen)
   2. collect a list of current medications (medication reconciliation)
   3. ask focused questions about the client's support system and explore social issues (housing, access to food, financial status, etc.)

See chapter 2 for more information on the qualifications and scope of practice for behavioral health professionals.

The following definitions may assist the behavioral case manager with motivational interviewing, planning, and implementing care:

+ **addiction**: dependence on a substance or practice that is physically or psychologically habit forming to the extent that critical pain and damage results
+ **adverse consequences**: unwanted outcome as the result of engaging in harmful physical, psychological, or social practices
+ **behavioral health care**: care focused on the diagnosis and treatment of behavioral health issues
+ **dual diagnosis**: having more than one diagnosis
+ **self-neglect**: the practice of harming oneself by refusing to care for one's self appropriately
+ **severe and persistent mental illness (SPMI)**: often defined as the most critical and devastating form of mental illness and is known to cause permanent disturbances in thoughts, emotions, and relationships with the world
+ **substance abuse**: the continued use of a medication without medical reason; excessive and intentional use of a controlled substance (alcohol, narcotics, etc.)
+ **substance dependence**: a deep physical and/or psychological need to use a controlled substance to achieve a feeling of euphoria and/or calmness
+ **substance use**: the nonmedically warranted consumption of medications or substances such as tobacco, alcohol, or illicit drugs

PRACTICE QUESTION

6. Which of the following best describes substance abuse?
    A) the unwarranted, intentional, and continual use of a substance
    B) the deep need to use a substance to achieve a particular feeling
    C) excessive but sporadic use of a substance
    D) the use of a controlled substance while not under the care of a doctor

ABUSE AND NEGLECT

Case managers often manage clients who have endured one or more types of abuse and/or neglect. Types of abuse or neglect include:

+ **neglect**: the failure or refusal to appropriately care for someone
+ **abuse**: the brutal and sadistic treatment of an individual
+ **emotional abuse**: a pattern of controlling, negative behavior that can include criticism, shaming, name calling, withholding affection, isolation, or refusing to communicate

+ **emotional neglect**: the failure to acknowledge another's feelings or to intentionally withhold affection

+ **psychological abuse**: tormenting an individual through manipulation to do certain things, usually affecting one's inner thoughts and feelings

+ **physical abuse**: intentionally hurting someone (hitting, punching, kicking), typically repeatedly

+ **financial (or economic) abuse**: when an individual acquires and maintains control over another's access to financial resources

The signs and symptoms of abuse and neglect vary greatly and depend on the type of abuse suffered. Survivors of physical abuse may exhibit heavy guarding of their own anatomy; flinch at sudden, unexpected movements; and will likely have sustained physical injuries that are in various stages of healing. Those who have experienced emotional abuse and/or neglect have been made to feel worthless. They may avoid sharing their feelings and innermost desires. They may isolate themselves, self-criticize, and self-deprecate.

Encouraging an abuse survivor to discuss his or her issues can take time and patience. The most vital thing a case manager can do when managing these clients is to establish a rapport early on and be *very* patient and sensitive. Those who experience abuse may not be eager to talk about it and must be given ample time to trust and feel safe.

Once the client has divulged the details of the abuse, it is up to the case manager to first ensure that the client is safe. If the client is in danger, the CCM must contact authorities and should help remove the client from the environment. The client should be moved to a safe place away from the abuser, and the abuser should not know or be able to discover the client's whereabouts. Case managers usually have access to community resources such as shelters and housing for battered individuals, as well as direct contact information for a myriad of mental and emotional health care professionals. Once the client is safe, the case manager can work to ensure that the client is ready and willing to receive needed medical care and therapy.

PRACTICE QUESTION

7. Peter is an eight-year-old boy who presents to the ED with a broken arm. The ED case manager notices that this is Peter's fourth ED visit in three weeks. Upon further review of the chart, the case manager also notices that every time Peter has presented to the ED, his chief complaint is that he fell. Peter also has bruises on his inner forearms and upper arms, and his bottom lip is swollen. Based on these findings, the CCM believes that Peter is being subjected to physical abuse. What should be the case manager's next step?

   A) ignore these findings

   B) contact the local police department

   C) contact Child Protective Services (CPS)

   D) speak with the ED physician

END-OF-LIFE ISSUES

End-of-life discussions bring about difficult decisions. When managing end-of-life care, one must consider what the client wants or would have wanted, the client's power of attorney or advanced medical directive, and ethical considerations as they apply to both. **Hospice facilities** provide a comforting, stimulation-free environment that attends to a dying client's emotional and spiritual needs. **Palliative care** functions to make the client at the end of life more comfortable and as pain-free as possible to improve the quality of his or her remaining time.

> 🔍 Case managers can be instrumental in helping a client's loved ones prepare for their passing by assisting with arrangements to memorialize the client and allowing time for loved ones to grieve.

Caring for the client at the end of life can be challenging for the caregiver as well as the client's family. Contemplating withdrawal of care and adhering to a Do Not Resuscitate (DNR) order is usually painful for the loved ones, as they are struggling with the possibility of recovery, quality of life, and what the patient's wishes are. This time is especially tense if the family is large and torn between what they desire and what the patient desires. It is important for health care professionals and the client's case manager to be sensitive to the family's needs and desires as well as the client's, while also giving the family private time to grieve and discuss options.

PRACTICE QUESTION

8. Tina has stage-four breast cancer and is currently being cared for in a hospice facility. Which question is *most* appropriate for the case manager to discuss with Tina and her family regarding end-of-life decisions?

    A) "How would you prefer to be remembered?"

    B) "Do you have an advanced directive or power of attorney?"

    C) "Have you chosen a funeral home yet?"

    D) "When would you like to discuss your options and desires for end-of-life care?"

CHRONIC ILLNESS AND DISABILITY

The case manager managing a client who has a chronic illness or disability has many factors to consider, such as multiple comorbidities, alternative therapies and interventions, and the client's frame of mind. The CCM must also update the plan of care as new developments arise and keep in close contact with professionals of all disciplines consulting on the client's case. Case managers must be understanding and patient, and they should allow clients to verbalize their thoughts about their conditions, treatments, and anticipated results.

It can be especially difficult to care for the client with multiple chronic health conditions, as a care plan must be formulated for each diagnosis that addresses the client's physical, mental, and emotional needs and goals. An emotional setback can hinder physical progress, so the client must be made aware of any changes or developments in the plan of care and be permitted to express fears openly. Remaining in self-directed care promotes stable emotional and mental health.

PRACTICE QUESTION

9. A case manager is caring for a client with type 2 diabetes and chronic hypertension. How would the case manager *best* start a conversation with the client to assess how she feels about her health care experience?

    A) "Would you like to tell me what you're thinking and feeling about your care?"

    B) "I'd like for you to tell me how you feel about your treatment."

    C) "Is there something you want to tell me about your care?"

    D) "Would you like me to tell you more about your treatment options?"

SELF-HARM AND SUICIDE

Case managers may have clients who have a history of or who are threatening self-harm or suicide. **Self-harm** is the intentional infliction of injury on one's own body. Common forms of self-harm include cutting and burning. **Suicide** is intentionally causing one's own death. Risk factors for suicide include behavioral health disorders like depression and bipolar disorder; a history of trauma or abuse; and environmental stressors like bullying, divorce, or job loss. People who have previously attempted suicide are at a much higher risk for suicide attempts.

When managing clients who are at risk of self-harm or suicide, the case manager needs to build trust and develop a rapport with the client. As the relationship grows, the client will hopefully feel comfortable enough to divulge relevant information about his or her emotional and mental history, which can provide the case manager with some insight into causes of current behavior. Once the case manager has the most detailed picture available, the CCM can begin to develop a plan of care to address the self-harm and underlying issues.

If a case manager is speaking to a client over the phone who is threatening to harm him- or herself, the case manager must keep the client on the phone while alerting another individual who can dial 911. Distressed callers are never to be allowed off the phone, nor are they to be placed on hold.

Similarly, during a field visit, the case manager can call authorities or a behavioral health facility for mobile evaluation of a client who is a danger to him- or herself. No permission is needed for the evaluation, but in most cases the client cannot be forced to accept care. Clients must be informed of the option to see a mental health professional, but barring extreme circumstances, the decision is up to the client. A case manager must be prepared for the possibility that some clients may react with hostility. The best recourse is to remain calm, understanding, and not take personal offense.

PRACTICE QUESTION

10. What is the LEAST appropriate thing a case manager can say to a client who is on the phone and threatening to take his own life?

    A) "I am here to help you."

    B) "Calm down so I can understand you."

    C) "I understand that you are having a difficult time right now."

    D) "Please talk to me and tell me how you feel."

CRISIS INTERVENTION STRATEGIES

Crisis intervention is defined as the immediate psychotherapy during an acute critical situation with the intent of restoring the individual to a pre-crisis level of functioning. Examples of a crisis include natural disasters, death of a loved one, physical injury, or combative behavior.

Case managers often must grapple with the best and most effective way to speak with a client in a severe depressive episode or one who wishes to end his or her own life. Active listening is key. The case manager must absorb the client's words, understand what the client is expressing, and sympathize with the client.

Crisis intervention focuses on employing short-term approaches to prevent damages or injuries. One such approach is educating clients about typical responses to abnormal situations and reassuring them that their reactions to the crisis are short lived. Crisis intervention is often followed by long-term therapy to promote psychological health and well-being.

PRACTICE QUESTION

11. Crisis intervention is composed of all of the following elements EXCEPT

A) active listening

B) immediate action

C) long-term care

D) education

Psychosocial Support Systems
WELLNESS AND ILLNESS PREVENTION PROGRAMS

Strategies for preventing illness and promoting wellness are instrumental in helping case managers formulate goals for care plans. Many factors that contribute to the development of serious illnesses are often **modifiable**, meaning they are within one's control. For example, eating a healthy, well-balanced diet and exercising regularly can help prevent illnesses like type 2 diabetes, hypertension, and obesity in many individuals.

Several managed care health maintenance organizations (HMOs) and preferred provider organizations (PPOs) have case management departments. These departments focus on wellness and illness prevention or give clients the tools they need to self-manage their conditions to prevent complications. Furthermore, many insurance companies provide incentives to clients who keep all scheduled physicians' appointments, report relevant lab data, and refill medications as ordered. These incentives range from gift cards to reduced insurance premiums.

PRACTICE QUESTION

12. Which of the following is a modifiable risk factor for developing hypertension?

A) age

B) race

C) diet

D) gender

SUPPORT PROGRAMS

The purpose of **support programs** is to provide aid to those in need of comfort and guidance in living with challenging conditions. Support programs often take the form of discussion groups. They are typically facilitated by counselors or by other individuals who have directly experienced the situation that the support group addresses. For example, Alcoholics Anonymous meetings are conducted by recovering alcoholics.

Support groups are conducted this way for several reasons. First, it is considered more effective to have a facilitator whose wisdom and experience can be a benefit to others. Secondly, the facilitator can also defuse controversy and make sure everyone gets a turn to speak. In addition, this arrangement allows a judgment-free environment, since everyone in attendance has had similar experiences. Finally, support groups are generally voluntary; members attend for their own benefit.

> While attending support groups is usually voluntary, in some cases it is legally mandated. For instance, attending a certain number of Alcoholics Anonymous or Narcotics Anonymous meetings might be part of an offender's sentence.

There are many common support groups that can be found in most communities. These include Alcoholics Anonymous (AA), Narcotics Anonymous (NA), Gamblers Anonymous (GA), grief and bereavement counseling groups, groups for those who have survived abuse and/or sexual violence, and groups that support members with chronic illnesses like diabetes or Crohn's disease, to name just a few. Support groups also exist for the families of people with issues such as alcoholism or cancer, and for families who have lost members to violence or suicide.

PRACTICE QUESTION

13. Which of these is NOT an element of support groups?

A) the facilitator determines if participants can join the support group

B) participants are there voluntarily because they want to heal

C) all participants share a common experience

D) the facilitator may have experienced the condition

COMMUNITY RESOURCES

Community resources exist to enhance the life quality of those who reside in the community. A resource of this type can be a person, building or structure, community service or business. Eldercare services, for example, can provide meals to the elderly, help them maintain the structural integrity of their homes, and have trusted professionals and community volunteers come to the home to perform chores.

> Pastoral counseling integrates a faith-based perspective and spiritual guidance with psychology. It is offered by a trained minister or other clergyperson. Clients who attend religious institutions may have access to this service.

Religious organizations such as missions and youth groups serve the community via soup kitchens, clothing/toy donation drives, and mission projects that may involve building houses for the homeless or providing medical care to the indigent. **Government programs** often provide financial aid for communities, whether it be Medicaid, assistance through the Department of Housing and Urban Development (HUD), or grants and scholarships for school. **Meal delivery programs** such as Meals on Wheels and Nurture Life deliver meals to the elderly and children, respectively. **Pharmacy assistance programs** offer medication prescriptions at discounted rates, which is an excellent resource for the elderly who have been prescribed multiple medications and are on a fixed budget.

PRACTICE QUESTION

14.   What is the main goal of community resources?

    A)   enhance the quality of life for community members

    B)   provide meals and medical care to members of the community

    C)   build homes for the homeless in the community

    D)   deliver meals to members of the community

HEALTH COACHING

The purpose and process of **health coaching** is to inspire health behavior change through evidence-based conversation, education, and clinical strategies designed to improve health and wellness. As with any type of case or care management, this process involves establishing and fostering a positive and trusting relationship with the individual, completing a detailed health assessment, and developing a plan of care—often referred to as a wellness vision.

The creation of the wellness vision is collaborative and focuses on the strengths of the individual, what he or she would like to accomplish, and steps to achieve goals. A case manager's role is similar to the role of a health coach. Both professions motivate and inspire the client to create a positive change through behavior modification to improve overall health.

15. The wellness vision developed by an individual and health coach does all of the following EXCEPT

    A) center on desired results

    B) concentrate on deadlines

    C) focus on steps to achieve goals

    D) concentrate on strengths and weaknesses

Family Dynamics

A **family dynamic** is how members of a family communicate and relate to each another. How a client interacts with his or her family plays a large role in the success of case management of that client. A strong support system is integral to the achievement of goals and fosters improved well-being.

When a case manager conducts an initial interview, great care is taken to discuss the client's support system. Such inquiries may include:

+ Do you live alone?

+ Are you married or in a committed partnership?

+ Do you have children?

+ How would you characterize your relationship with your significant other/ children/other members of your family?

The case manager may also conduct a **home visit** to observe the family dynamic firsthand. Focused questions and direct observation paint a detailed picture of how the client's family members function as individuals and as a cohesive unit. With an understanding of a client's relationship with his or her family, the CCM can explore how that relationship can support the plan of care to result in positive outcomes.

PRACTICE QUESTION

16. Sarah is a seventeen-year-old female who is pregnant for the first time. You have been assigned as her perinatal case manager. What question might you ask her in the initial interview to learn more about her family's dynamic?

    A) "How did your parents react to your pregnancy, with you being so young?"

    B) "Are you and your babydaddy still involved?"

    C) "How does your family feel about your pregnancy?"

    D) "How do you get along with your family?"

Multicultural, Spiritual, and Religious Factors

Cultural, spiritual, and religious factors may affect a client's health status. These same factors can also affect client communication, compliance with treatment regimen, and support system. It is important for health care professionals to be cognizant of these factors when diagnosing and treating these individuals.

A person's identity can be directly tied to his or her culture and religious faith, so respect for these differences is integral to developing a plan of care. For example, many individuals who practice Islam or Judaism abstain from consuming pork, so other proteins would have to be discussed when formulating a meal plan. Race and ethnicity may also be considered, as they can determine a predisposition to certain illnesses and chronic conditions (i.e., African Americans are more prone to developing hypertension than people of other backgrounds).

Language barriers and different dialects play a huge part in whether the client can advocate for him- or herself, ask questions, and understand instructions. Some cultures' body language and expressions of anxiety may be indicative of a deeper problem within the family dynamic and should be explored with the client in private. To build trust and foster a symbiotic relationship, health care professionals should remain nonjudgmental when presented with cultural or spiritual beliefs that differ from their own.

Caregivers must understand the cultural and spiritual traditions of a host of diverse backgrounds. Annual cultural sensitivity training is usually required in most health care settings. Such training, as well as discussions about differing religious factors that affect how individuals respond to health care, establishes a more positive working relationship between the health care professional and client.

PRACTICE QUESTION

17. Sheila is a Chinese American woman giving birth to her second child. She is having contractions every two to three minutes but does little more than grimace with the pain, and she appears to be happy because she is smiling. What is the *most* appropriate conclusion that a well-trained health care professional could come to, given Sheila's behavior?

   A) "Sheila must not really be in that much pain because she is smiling."

   B) "Chinese Americans must not want to show weakness by screaming or crying out."

   C) "Sheila must not know what it means to be in pain, or she has never felt severe physical pain."

   D) "It is unlikely that Sheila's response to pain is related to her ethnic background."

Communication Techniques

Interpersonal Communication

The theory of basic communication is made up of several components, which are defined below:

+ **sender**: the individual or thing sending the message
+ **channel**: the method by which the sender transmits the message
+ **receiver**: the individual or thing translating the message
+ **destination**: the individual or thing for whom the message is targeted
+ **message**: the information transferred from the sender to the recipient

People use these elements in everyday conversations without even realizing it. The sender will transfer information through the channel to the receiver, who interprets or translates the message to the destination. More recently, oral conversation has given way to texting, emailing, and using social media; sometimes the intended tone of the message risks being lost without aural cues.

Active listening means paying attention to the speaker, not just hearing their words. The listener makes eye contact with the speaker to indicate interest in what is being said. An active listener repeats important points the speaker has made to ensure understanding, asks follow-up questions, and does not interrupt. The goal is twofold: better understanding, and to make the speaker aware that the listener cares about what the speaker is saying.

The basic elements of communication and active listening form the foundation of a case manager's rapport and relationship with the client. To build a strong rapport with a client, the CCM must be engaging, an active listener, and avoid interrupting the client. Clients will trust that the CCM cares about their issues and advocates for their well-being. A case manager who actively listens and delivers on guarantees builds trust with the client. While building trust can take time, it makes managing the client's health condition easier for all involved.

PRACTICE QUESTION

18. Which of the following is NOT an example of active listening when working with a client?

    A) documenting findings on the computer during the visit

    B) expressing empathy when the client discusses her health issues

    C) making eye contact during the interview

    D) clarifying a client's statement that caused confusion

Conflict Resolution Strategies

Conflict resolution is important in the workplace and beyond. Some strategies to resolve conflict include conflict avoidance, giving in, standing one's ground, compromising, and collaborating.

Conflict avoidance involves not acknowledging the conflict. **Giving in** means acquiescing to the other party, thereby giving them what they want or letting them have their way. **Standing one's ground** is a way of competing with the opposing party in the hopes that they do not win the battle. **Compromising** involves seeking out common ground as a stepping stone to negotiating and resolving the conflict. **Collaborating** consists of actively listening to the opposing party's perspective, discussing areas of like-mindedness and common objectives, and confirming that both parties understand each other's viewpoint. This strategy is sometimes difficult but can be rewarding when it is effective.

PRACTICE QUESTION

19. Jolie is a manager of a case management department in a hospital. Mary, one of her employees, is constantly at odds with Nicole, another employee. Mary has seniority over Nicole but is not her direct superior. Mary wants Jolie to write Nicole up for disrespecting her. Jolie listens to both sides but takes no action, going on about her work as if no conflict has occurred. What type of conflict resolution strategy is Jolie employing?

A) compromising

B) conflict avoidance

C) giving in

D) collaboration

Answer Key

1. A) Incorrect. The contemplation stage occurs when the individual seriously thinks about changing a behavior and what steps may be involved.

   B) Correct. The precontemplation stage is when the individual is not thinking about behavioral change and not ready to take steps to change.

   C) Incorrect. The maintenance stage occurs after the action stage, when the individual has made the change in behavior and is trying to stick to it.

   D) Incorrect. The action stage is when the individual has performed the action to change the behavior.

2. A) Incorrect. While preparing to contact a client for an initial interview, the case manager will review recent hospitalizations, if any exist.

   B) Incorrect. The case manager will review the client's provider information.

   C) Correct. The case manager will not enter a UR request for the client, as she has not spoken to the client yet, and that is usually handled by a different department.

   D) Incorrect. The case manager will review any substance abuse history.

3. **D) Correct.** The NVS would be an appropriate tool to use, as it focuses on reading nutrition labels and is available in English and Spanish.

4. **A) Correct.** This behavior typifies a localized response. Eleanor is responding to stimuli, but the same stimuli produces a different reaction each time.

   B) Incorrect. Eleanor is not quite at the stage where she is aware of herself and family, which is indicative of the confused-appropriate stage of recovery.

   C) Incorrect. Eleanor is far from independently functioning within society, which is indicative of the purposeful-appropriate stage of recovery.

   D) Incorrect. No response would mean that Eleanor did not respond at all to the ice cube in her palm.

5. A) Incorrect. The CCM is delegating an important CCM task to the family member.

   B) Incorrect. Blood pressure monitors are bought over the counter and do not need a prescription.

   C) Incorrect. Simply providing a pamphlet on the importance of blood pressure monitoring is not likely to help Sam, who needs to learn how to acquire and use a monitor.

   D) Correct. Sam should speak with his insurance provider. Often there are benefits that help cover some or all of the cost of the monitor.

6. **A) Correct.** Abuse is the continual, intentional use of a substance without a medical reason.

   B) Incorrect. *Dependence* is the need to use a substance to achieve a desired effect.

C)   Incorrect. Substance abuse is continual, not sporadic.

D)   Incorrect. The definition of substance abuse does not address whether a person is under the care of a doctor.

7. A)   Incorrect. The case manager would not ignore these findings.

    B)   Incorrect. The case manager would not contact the local police department.

    C)   **Correct.** The case manager would contact CPS, as he or she has an obligation to report any suspected or known abuse of a child.

    D)   Incorrect. The case manager should notify the ED physician, but this would not be the immediate next step following the conclusion of abuse.

8. A)   Incorrect. This question is not the most appropriate question to ask at this time.

    B)   Incorrect. Advanced directive or power of attorney should already have been discussed, and the information should be in the client's file.

    C)   Incorrect. This question is completely inappropriate and insensitive. Furthermore, it may cause the client to feel resentment toward the case manager.

    D)   **Correct.** This is the correct and appropriate question to ask; the client and family should control the timing of unpleasant discussions.

9. **A)**   **Correct.** This question is inviting the client to verbalize concerns and allows her to decide how much she would like to share.

    B)   Incorrect. This statement is addressing what the case manager wants, not what the client wants.

    C)   Incorrect. This question assumes the client has a particular issue to discuss and does not explicitly offer the client a chance to share her feelings.

    D)   Incorrect. This question focuses on treatment options, not the client's feelings about her care, and does not offer the client the opportunity to share with the case manager.

10. A)   Incorrect. It is important to let the client know that someone is there to help them.

    B)   **Correct.** A case manager must never tell a client threatening to take his or her own life to "calm down." This expression invalidates the client's feelings. The client may hang up the phone.

    C)   Incorrect. Sympathizing with the client assures him that someone is listening to him and cares about his concerns and well-being.

    D)   Incorrect. Encouraging conversation about the client's feelings and thoughts will keep him talking—and not acting out on harmful impulses—while the case manager alerts another individual to call 911.

11. A)   Incorrect. Crisis intervention must involve active listening to get to the root of the issue.

    B)   Incorrect. Crisis intervention is immediate and is only meant to employ short-term strategies.

C) **Correct.** Crisis intervention is based on short-term goals, and long-term care often follows once the critical situation is defused.

D) Incorrect. Crisis intervention has an educational component to help individuals in crisis understand that a crisis—and the intense emotional reaction to it—is temporary.

12. A) Incorrect. Age is not a modifiable risk factor.

B) Incorrect. Race is not a modifiable risk factor.

C) **Correct.** Diet is within one's control and is therefore modifiable.

D) Incorrect. Gender is not a modifiable risk factor.

13. A) **Correct.** In most support groups, participants only need to show up—they do not need approval beforehand.

B) Incorrect. Most members of support groups want to be there to work on healing.

C) Incorrect. Support groups are built around a particular issue or experience (e.g., alcoholism) that participants share.

D) Incorrect. The facilitator of a support group is an individual who may have experienced what the support group focuses on.

14. A) **Correct.** The main goal of community resources is to improve the quality of life for those who live in the community. The other choices are part of this larger main goal.

15. A) Incorrect. The wellness vision will focus on desired results.

B) **Correct.** The vision will not concentrate on deadlines but will focus on an achievable time frame.

C) Incorrect. The vision will focus on steps to take in the goal-achievement process.

D) Incorrect. The wellness vision will concentrate on strengths as a means toward goal achievement.

16. A) Incorrect. This question is not appropriate to ask: it sounds judgmental and does not help to establish a rapport.

B) Incorrect. This question is inappropriately worded and therefore not an appropriate question to ask.

C) Incorrect. As a case manager, you are trying to discover what Sarah's relationship is with her family, not necessarily how her family feels about her.

D) **Correct.** This is an appropriate question, and it is open ended to allow for a more detailed response.

17. A) Incorrect. This is an incorrect assumption based on the client's different way of expressing pain.

B) Incorrect. This is an inappropriate and inaccurate statement with no foundation.

C) Incorrect. This statement could be viewed as insulting, as this is the client's second time giving birth.

D) **Correct.** This is the appropriate response; there is no reason to assume that Sheila's personal response to pain is necessarily related to her ethnic background.

18. **A)** **Correct.** Although computers are often used in the office or client's home, eye contact may be compromised, and the client may feel the CCM is not fully listening.

B) Incorrect. Expressing empathy is an important component of active listening.

C) Incorrect. Making eye contact is an important component of active listening.

D) Incorrect. Engaging with the content of the client's statements shows that the CCM is actively listening.

19. A) Incorrect. Jolie is not compromising, as she has listened to both sides but has not offered to facilitate negotiation or find any other resolution.

B) **Correct.** Jolie is practicing conflict avoidance; she is pretending that no conflict has happened.

C) Incorrect. Jolie is not giving in to Mary because she has not written Nicole up for anything.

D) Incorrect. Jolie *has* listened to both parties' perspectives, but she has not discussed areas of agreement or conflict resolution objectives with Mary or Nicole.

FIVE: QUALITY AND OUTCOMES EVALUATION AND MEASUREMENTS

Quality and Performance Improvement Concepts

Quality improvement is a formal approach to ensure that quality of care is achieved by providers and that they will conform to certain standards and guidelines. If a quality deficiency is detected, methods are designed to correct it and prevent future deficiencies.

Performance improvement refers to the study of the functioning of a health care organization to improve patient care. There are three types of measurements used to study performance:

+ **Process measurements** describe what occurs while care is given, with a focus on clinical guidelines. The percentage of patients who received vaccinations, for instance, is a process measurement.

+ **Structure measurements** describe how the care environment is structured. Staffing ratios are an example of a structure measurement.

+ **Outcome measurements** describe the result of patients' health care services. For example, mortality rates are outcome measurements.

Case managers collect performance improvement measurements through client surveys and call and documentation audits. These measurements develop performance improvement criteria to help case managers address problems.

> Performance improvement goals should be individualized. For example, a CCM might review her performance measurements and find that she takes an average of two hours to complete an initial assessment by telephone. Consequently, she might set a performance improvement goal to shorten assessment time.

1. Which performance improvement tactic might case managers use to enhance their time management skills?

    A) quickly reviewing a discharge summary with a recently discharged client

    B) examining the caseload for the day before start of shift

    C) skipping medication reconciliation on medications the client has taken before

    D) educating the client about his or her condition without allowing time for questions

Quality Indicators

TYPES OF QUALITY INDICATORS

A **quality indicator** is a measurement that gauges quality in health care operations. Creating and implementing quality indicators is vital to a case manager's position as a collaborative health coach and an integral member of the health care team. Such indicators must be developed using evidence-based criteria, quality assurance teams, and research to formulate the best tools, for these indicators will assist in evaluating outcomes for clients.

A **clinical indicator** is one that evaluates a health care organization's practices, methods, and results. One example is reviewing a skilled nursing facility's fall risk assessment and policies and procedures on patient safety.

A **financial indicator** measures cost and cost-effectiveness in relation to quality of health care delivered. For example, a managed health care organization may allot a certain amount of funds for fee-for-service (otherwise known as unbundling) and then compare that amount to the same services included in a covered plan to ascertain which is more prudent and which results in higher-quality outcomes.

Productivity indicators determine the amount of work being done. To calculate productivity, assign an average amount of time to a task and then compute how many hours of work an employee completed based on that estimation. For example, it takes two hours to complete an in-home initial assessment of a client and one hour to complete a follow-up assessment. If a case manager completed eight initial assessments and twenty follow-up assessments in one week, that case manager has achieved thirty-six hours of work in that week. Productivity indicators are useful in establishing the terms of a manageable caseload.

> Evidence-based practice refers to proven methods and processes that have yielded consistent outcomes. It is often the driving force behind productive case management; tried-and-true techniques achieve the most positive effects.

Utilization indicators reveal which services are the most used and if the frequent utilization of these services results in better outcomes for clients. A **utilization review** is a tool that determines the medical necessity of procedures, tests, and lab work. A team of utilization review nurses, physicians, and medical directors checks submitted clinical information to establish a basis of medical necessity contingent upon diagnosis and evidence-based practice. In this way, only medically necessary practices are compensated.

Client experience indicators allow the client to rate the health care service experience, including the case manager and case management encounter. This provides invaluable feedback to an organization or agency about its practices from a consumer's perspective. An example of this is a satisfaction survey, which presents questions about the friendliness, helpfulness, and overall efficiency of the case management program.

PRACTICE QUESTION

2. Documentation of a client's non-emergent hospital admission has been submitted to the client's insurance company by the provider. Who would initially assess for medical necessity?

    A) claims examiner

    B) medical director

    C) utilization review nurse

    D) financial analyst

QUALITY INDICATORS TECHNIQUES AND APPLICATIONS

Data on quality can be obtained in several different ways: reviewing client surveys, providers' care, and efficacy of case management as it relates to desired client outcomes. These techniques are typically used by a **quality assurance (QA) team** for reporting and statistical purposes and, most importantly, to assess where process change may be needed for improvement.

The **Plan, Do, Check, Act (PDCA)** method evaluates the outcome of a process for just that purpose. A *plan* is devised to solve a problem, that plan is implemented (*done*), the outcome of the implemented action is reexamined (*checked*), and a new plan is formulated to address and overcome the obstacle that the original plan revealed (*act*).

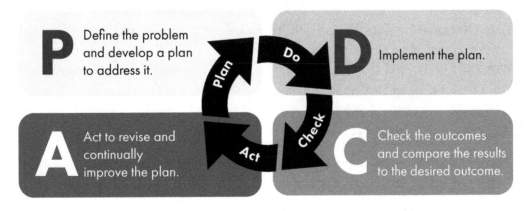

Figure 5.1. Plan, Do, Check, Act (PDCA)

Another useful technique used in quality improvement is the **lean approach.** This method endorses the process of constant, small changes being made in routines and practices to enhance value and effectiveness.

PRACTICE QUESTION

3. During which phase of PDCA would the QA team meet to discuss ways to facilitate a better method of case manager–client interaction?

A) Do

B) Act

C) Check

D) Plan

SOURCES OF QUALITY INDICATORS

Many agencies and organizations help to establish standards of care and quality through their mission statements and accreditation processes. One such organization is the **Centers for Medicare and Medicaid Services (CMS).** This group administers and regulates standards of practice and quality for Medicare, Medicaid, the Children's Health Insurance Program (CHIP), and the Health Insurance Marketplace. Its central mission is to provide high-quality and affordable health care.

The **Utilization Review Accreditation Commission (URAC)** authorizes the processes and practices of the agencies and organizations that deliver medical care services. Any health care organization undergoing URAC review must initially obtain core accreditation—adherence to basic URAC standards. Core accreditation is required for subsequent URAC accreditation programs.

 Accrediting bodies and other agencies and organizations are constantly molding and shaping the standards of health care in our world.

Another agency is the **National Committee for Quality Assurance (NCQA),** which relies heavily on evidence-based standards to govern and enrich the care provided by health care plans. The **National Quality Forum (NQF)** measures quality by supporting and enhancing client safety, as well as realizing improved client outcomes. Finally, the **Agency for Healthcare Research and Quality (AHRQ)** uses research and experimentation to determine the suitability of health care services and access to care.

PRACTICE QUESTION

4. Which technique is NOT used by organizations that monitor quality?

A) studying protected health information

B) relying on evidence-based standards

C) granting accreditation to health care organizations

D) conducting research and experimentation

Accreditation Standards and Requirements

Accreditation is a process by which an organization or agency receives or earns credentials. These credentials are indicators of exceptional performance and quality. With accreditation, an organization can expand its client base, meet state and federal regulatory requirements, and distinguish itself from competing organizations. Two main accreditation organizations are the Utilization Review Accreditation Commission (URAC) and the National Committee for Quality Assurance (NCQA), discussed in the previous section.

URAC accreditation demonstrates an entity's commitment to quality in delivering care. If a group or organization is URAC accredited, any business it conducts is consistent with national health care standards. Obtaining URAC accreditation is a lengthy and arduous process; just applying for accreditation can take anywhere from six to nine months.

As stated earlier, any health care agency undergoing URAC review must first obtain core accreditation before seeking any other accreditation. URAC offers a wide variety of accreditation programs in topics like dental and health plans, disease management, and case management. Each area possesses its own standards and criteria for accreditation.

 URAC accreditation is often referred to as the "gold standard" of all accreditations, as it is widely considered to represent excellence in quality health care delivery.

NCQA offers certification to entities that provide specialized services, and accreditation to groups that offer services that are more inclusive. One of the main tools NCQA employs is the Healthcare Effectiveness and Data Information Set (HEDIS), which specifically assesses quality of performance as it relates to standards of care and service. This agency also uses Consumer Assessment of Healthcare Providers and Systems (CAHPS) data by gathering relevant client survey information from health plans and providers, as well as conducting comprehensive research on such topics as client-centered care and innovations in quality measurement.

Another major health care accrediting body is the **Joint Commission**, which evaluates the processes and practices of health care organizations to ensure that they are providing the highest quality of affordable care. The Joint Commission offers accreditation to hospitals, home care agencies, and other providers. It also offers certification to health care staffing services and primary care medical homes.

PRACTICE QUESTION

5. Which of the following is NOT a reason for an agency or organization to seek accreditation?

    A)   increase its credibility

    B)   distinguish itself from the competition

    C)   gain more control over pricing

    D)   meet regulatory requirements

Data Interpretation and Reporting

Reviewing and reporting data requires a knowledge of basic data terminology. **Validity** refers to the meaningfulness of the data; in other words, whether the data is measuring what it is supposed to be measuring. **Accurate** data is data that is correct or true. **Reliability**, with regard to a scientific demonstration, means that the same experiment conducted repeatedly would have the same outcome each time.

Data can be used to determine case manager productivity and care quality, which is important in reporting outcomes. Data reporting for case managers is designed to show that the case manager's interventions improved patient outcomes. Case managers may be asked to provide data related to patient care reports, for quality improvement, to justify continuing services, and to show the benefits of having a case manager.

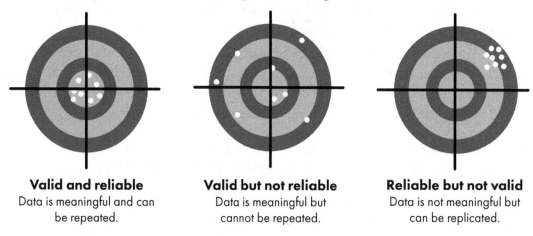

Valid and reliable
Data is meaningful and can be repeated.

Valid but not reliable
Data is meaningful but cannot be repeated.

Reliable but not valid
Data is not meaningful but can be replicated.

Figure 5.2. Reliability and Validity

But how can data best be interpreted and applied? For example, in remote case management, or case management conducted by phone, positive outcomes may be correlated with the number of contact attempts made. The case manager may then determine that, to be more successful and assist clients with achieving optimum results, he or she must increase call volume. The next step in that process would be to increase call volume with other clients and search for similarities (reliability) among all client findings.

Case management managers or directors may also attempt to justify the expansion of a case management department by hiring additional employees. To support their argument, they might present data showing the number of clients awaiting case management services plus the number of clients already in case management, divided by the number of employees.

Call and documentation **audits** play a role in quality improvement; the quality of a call or documentation can be connected to more positive outcomes for a client. Such audits would be used in quality improvement reports and possibly even to formulate a corrective action plan for a case manager who is struggling.

6. How might a case manager determine that a client's enrollment in an asthma case management program has been successful?

    A) The client has attended all his grandson's baseball games.

    B) The client has stopped refilling his medications.

    C) The client has had more acute visits to the pulmonologist.

    D) The client has reported increased exposure to asthma triggers.

Health Care Analytics

HEALTH RISK ASSESSMENT

A case manager may gather information from a client-completed **health risk assessment (HRA)** to determine the medical, social, and educational needs of the client. This assessment will allow the case manager to evaluate the client's complete health picture to formulate and execute a plan of care. The HRA may elicit demographic data (age and gender), relevant medical history and surgeries, current illnesses and medications, any behavioral or emotional health issues (depression or anxiety), social support, and habits (alcohol and substance use or smoking).

The assessment can be completed in one of three ways: in person, by phone, or by the client online. There are disadvantages to self-reporting the HRA, however. The client may not wish to be completely honest, misunderstand the questions, or struggle with literacy or language comprehension. Performing the evaluation in person, the case manager can address some of these obstacles. An in-person evaluation also allows the case manager to assess the client's living conditions. The CCM should pay close attention to health hazards within the home (mold, loose rugs or carpeting, faulty electric wiring) and possible barriers to care like unreliable transportation or distance from the provider's office.

Once the case manager has contacted the client, there are certain actions that must be taken to establish a rapport:

+ Greet the client, provide an introduction, and explain the reason for the call or visit.
+ Ask the client how they are doing.
+ Allow the client time to answer questions and discuss the situation.
+ Discuss client-centered goals.
+ Use plain language, avoiding medical jargon to ensure client understanding.
+ Encourage questions and address any concerns; remain helpful.
+ Let the client know when the next phone call or home visit will occur.
+ Thank the client for their time.

HRAs are typically obtained by the primary care physician. The Affordable Care Act specifies that the HRA is part of the wellness exam for Medicare beneficiaries, and HRAs are also used for Medicaid enrollment.

PRACTICE QUESTION

7. Which of the following would NOT be considered relevant health risk assessment information from an elderly female client?

   A) how often she takes her medication

   B) her feelings about her illnesses and her current support system

   C) the name of the pediatrician she saw as a child

   D) how many meals and snacks she eats daily

PREDICTIVE MODELING

Predictive modeling uses numerical or statistical data to forecast results. It is primarily used to anticipate the likelihood of an outcome when a specific set of data is entered into the equation. This modeling is useful to determine whether an individual will have frequent hospitalizations due to a high-risk disease. If the model forecasts they are at high risk for repeated hospitalization, a case manager's services may be used to help reduce the number of visits.

For example, a case manager may want to determine the risk of hospitalization for a pregnant client with a history of pregnancy-induced hypertension (PIH). The case manager must consider several factors:

   ✦ the outcome of a previous pregnancy when PIH was also present

   ✦ the client's history of multidisciplinary care (for instance, meeting with a hematologist and a maternal-fetal medicine specialist) throughout a previous pregnancy versus during the current pregnancy

   ✦ the client's current medication regimen, if any

   ✦ the client's compliance with the current plan of care

Case managers perform predictive modeling so often that it becomes second nature. It is essential to outcome management and reporting. To thoroughly complete the process, a client's comprehensive medical history must be available for review to determine patterns of behavior, provider recommendations, and outcomes of previous interventions. A case manager must think of a client's medical history as the beginning of a story that is still being told, and the goal is a "happily ever after" ending.

PRACTICE QUESTION

8. A case manager uses predictive modeling to assess the risk of hospitalization for a client with adult-onset diabetes. Which of the following factors is MOST important for the case manager to consider?

   A) childhood visit to neurologist for headaches

   B) previous HgbA1C result

   C) family history of hypertension

   D) current marital status

Adjusted Clinical Group (ACG)

The School of Public Health at Johns Hopkins University developed the **Adjusted Clinical Group system** (www.cmbodyofknowledge.com) to predict and compare the incidence of illness among similar groups of individuals. This establishes the most reasonable way to assess adequate provider functioning, assist with identifying clients at higher-than-normal risk, and foresee increased frequency of provider office visits, emergency department visits, urgent care facility visits, and hospitalizations. Essentially, this system is a more broad-based form of predictive modeling; it compiles and analyzes data from a larger group of people.

PRACTICE QUESTION

9. The results of an Adjusted Clinical Group study can help to determine all the following EXCEPT

    A) increased probability of certain members of the group to develop congestive heart failure (CHF).

    B) resemblances in how providers formulate a plan of care.

    C) who in the group is most likely to experience the loss of a child.

    D) how many people in the group will visit the emergency department more than twice in a year.

Caseload Calculation

Caseload Calculation is the process by which a caseload is computed. The following factors are considered in caseload calculation:

+ client acuity
+ risk stratification
+ case management setting (remote/by phone or onsite)
+ type of care management program (short term or long term)
+ role, expertise, and training of the case manager
+ supervisory controls
+ type of documentation used (paper or computerized)
+ other professional responsibilities

The Case Management Society of America (CMSA) developed a **Caseload Capacity Calculator** to determine what constitutes an accurate and realistic caseload, based on the variables listed above. Average caseload can also be determined by analyzing results from surveys taken by case managers, which may make the following queries:

+ What is your typical caseload broken down by day? By week?
+ How does case status contribute to your caseload? Is more time usually spent performing an initial assessment as compared to a follow-up assessment?

- Do specific case management programs yield a higher number of clients?
- How does client population affect your caseload?

Unfortunately, there is no one true answer to what represents a standard caseload, because there are so many elements to consider.

PRACTICE QUESTION

10. A team lead in case management performs many of the duties of a supervisor, like auditing, development and implementation of process improvement, and so on. At the same time, the team lead manages a caseload. Based on this information, which of the following would be accurate?

    A) A team lead should have as many cases as the other case managers.

    B) A team lead should have more cases than the other case managers.

    C) A team lead should have no cases at all.

    D) A team lead should have fewer cases than the other case managers.

Cost-Benefit Analysis

Case managers can use a **cost-benefit report** to determine or predict the monetary outcome of an action. **Hard savings** are current dollars saved and are directly related to the case manager's actions. For example, when patients are transferred to a lower level of acuity, or the length of their hospital stay is decreased, less money will be spent on and by the patient.

 Use the following formula to calculate hard or soft savings: savings = predicted cost – actual cost.

Soft savings are potential dollars saved in the future. Fewer and shorter hospitalizations, decreased need for durable medical equipment and supplies, and reduction in the use of home health services all result in soft savings. For example, consider a diabetic patient with a history of multiple visits to the ED. When the case manager takes on the client, she begins to diligently educate the client about diet, exercise, carbohydrate counting, and compliance with insulin self-administration. The case manager also maintains continual contact with the client's endocrinologist and primary care physician. Thanks to the case manager's work, the client has not had another visit to the ED. The soft savings are the money that would have been spent on the ED visit.

PRACTICE QUESTION

11. A case manager is managing a thirty-eight-weeks pregnant client who has diabetes. Her previous pregnancy ended in the delivery of an infant at thirty-three weeks gestation, who remained in the NICU for seven weeks. If the client were to deliver within the next twenty-four hours, and the infant was not admitted to the NICU, how would cost savings be calculated?

A) cost of one NICU day multiplied by the number of days previous infant was in the NICU

B) cost of one NICU day divided by the number of days previous infant was in the NICU

C) cost of one NICU day rounded down, then multiplied by the number of days previous infant was in the NICU

D) cost of all the NICU days combined and divided by thirty

Program Evaluation and Research Methods

Case managers work tirelessly to help clients manage their conditions and promote healthy outcomes. They want to feel assured that their efforts are not wasted, and **program evaluation** helps to determine and spotlight the achievements of case management. With more emphasis on outcome management and reporting, case managers must realize the value of their work and strive to continually improve processes and practices.

Client satisfaction surveys are one way to measure the efficacy and success of a case management program. A client will be asked a series of questions about his or her case manager (friendliness, timeliness of interactions, helpfulness), and about the case management program in general (client experience of specific program elements, best aspect, worst aspect, how to improve, and so on). These findings will usually be analyzed by a QA team, with feedback provided to the case manager and his or her direct supervisor. Case management outcomes can be gauged by monthly reporting of **success stories**. These stories normally are recorded in a standard format, covering the issue(s), the action or intervention taken, and the outcome.

With each case manager completing several evaluations a month, the evidence for case management grows. Success stories highlight the value of case management, especially when they are accompanied by cost-savings analysis and comparison charts showing positive outcomes experienced by clients. These calculations measure the success of case management programs and make the results clear to supervisors and institutions.

PRACTICE QUESTION

12. What type of question is NOT likely to appear on a client satisfaction survey?

A) How often did your case manager contact you?

B) Was your case manager friendly and helpful?

C) What is your marital status?

D) On a scale from 1 – 10, with 1 being poor and 10 being excellent, how would you rate your case management experience?

Answer Key

1. **A)** Incorrect. Upon transition of care, especially from hospital to home, the CCM should thoroughly review the discharge summary with the client and allow time for questions and further explanation, if necessary. If a client does not understand the discharge instructions, the client could end up back in the hospital.

   B) Correct. Examining a caseload before the start of a shift helps the case manager understand how busy the day will be. The CCM can work at a steady pace to maintain a productive, but not overburdened, workflow.

   C) Incorrect. Even if a client has taken a medication before, it is important to review the following: medication, dosage, frequency, route of administration, reason for medication, possible side effects, and adverse reactions. The client may have not taken the medication for some time and forgotten some details.

   D) Incorrect. One of a case manager's main responsibilities is to educate clients about their health conditions. A case manager who does not allow time for questions or feedback may mistakenly assume that the client understands a situation.

2. **A)** Incorrect. The claims examiner does not review clinical information; he or she processes the claim once it is submitted.

   B) Incorrect. The medical director will review the information only if the utilization review nurse submits the request for medical review.

   C) Correct. The utilization review nurse is the first-line responder to authorization requests and will review the clinical information once it is submitted by the provider or facility.

   D) Incorrect. Financial analysts do not review clinical information; they review expenditures and assess areas of financial liability.

3. **A)** Incorrect. The *Do* phase is also known as the implementation phase. Discussing a plan is not implementing a plan.

   B) Incorrect. The *Act* phase is the last component of PDCA. It consists of creating a new process to address the issues revealed during the "check" phase.

   C) Incorrect. The *Check* phase, which occurs after the plan has been implemented, evaluates the outcome of the plan.

   D) Correct. The initial *Plan* phase normally involves discussing how to resolve an issue.

4. **A) Correct.** Agencies that conduct accreditation reviews and monitor quality do not access protected health information as a part of their process.

   B) Incorrect. The NCQA uses evidence-based standards, among other criteria, to measure the quality of care delivered by health care plans.

   C) Incorrect. Both the NCQA and URAC are accrediting bodies and employ extensive processes to evaluate the quality of health care.

D) Incorrect. The AHRQ focuses on research and experiment results to ascertain which practices are relevant and which ones are obsolete.

5. A) Incorrect. Increasing the organization's credibility is an important reason to seek accreditation.

   B) Incorrect. Accreditation helps to set an organization apart from the others.

   C) Correct. Accreditation does not directly affect an organization's pricing structure.

   D) Incorrect. Many organizations will need to become accredited to meet regulatory requirements.

6. **A) Correct.** A client who has mismanaged asthma would be less likely to attend outdoor sporting events.

   B) Incorrect. Decreased frequency of medication refill shows that the client has not been thoroughly educated about the importance of refilling all medications in a timely manner.

   C) Incorrect. If a client is visiting his pulmonologist more frequently, he has most likely not been fully educated about controlling his condition. If his condition were under control, the visits would not be necessary.

   D) Incorrect. If a client reports increased or more frequent exposure to asthma triggers, he most likely has not been comprehensively educated about reduction of exposure to triggers, or he may be noncompliant due to lack of education from his case manager.

7. A) Incorrect. Medication reconciliation is a necessary part of the health risk assessment and helps to assess the client's knowledge of her medication(s).

   B) Incorrect. A client's feelings about her illnesses or conditions provides the case manager with insight into possible barriers to compliance, as well as her emotional status.

   C) Correct. The client's pediatrician when she was a child is not relevant; it is not pertinent to current conditions.

   D) Incorrect. Inquiring about meals and snacks provides the case manager with information about the client's nutritional status, eating habits, and access to certain foods.

8. A) Incorrect. While a case manager needs to know why a client visited a neurologist as a child, it is not the most important factor to consider in a diabetic patient.

   B) Correct. To help determine the current risk for a diabetic client, it is necessary to know the most recent HgbA1C result.

   C) Incorrect. While a family history of hypertension would be one factor to consider, it would not be the most important.

   D) Incorrect. The client's marital status is not relevant to the client's condition or plan of care.

9. A) Incorrect. The likelihood of the development of CHF in certain members of the group can be determined by conducting an ACG study, as one of the study's main purposes is to predict the incidence of illness, given a set of criteria.

B) Incorrect. ACG studies use information about shared practices within a provider specialty and compare how providers formulate care plans.

C) Correct. How likely a group member is to experience the loss of a child is not one of the criteria measured by an ACG study.

D) Incorrect. Using the data collected in the study, an ACG study can ascertain who will visit the ED, if the study defines the criteria for that outcome.

10. A) Incorrect. Because the team lead has also taken on supervisory duties, it is not appropriate that he or she have as many cases as the other case managers.

B) Incorrect. A team lead should not have more cases than the rest of the case managers, as he or she is responsible for other duties as well as case management.

C) Incorrect. A team lead is often expected to maintain a caseload, so having no cases at all is not appropriate.

D) Correct. A team lead should have a reasonable caseload to manage but fewer cases than the rest of the case managers because of other duties.

11. **A) Correct.** The cost of one NICU day multiplied by forty-nine days (number of days previous infant was in the NICU) would give the amount of money spent for the child's NICU stay. Because that cost has been avoided during this pregnancy, that cost represents soft savings.

12. A) Incorrect. Client satisfaction surveys will often elicit information about the frequency of case manager interaction to anticipate successful outcomes.

B) Incorrect. The survey will ask about a case manager's friendliness/helpfulness to determine how a rapport is developed.

C) Correct. Marital status is not relevant data on a client satisfaction survey and has no bearing on whether the case management program was successful.

D) Incorrect. Providing a rating scale helps to ascertain if a client would participate again in a case management program.

SIX: REHABILITATION CONCEPTS AND STRATEGIES

Vocational and Rehabilitation Service Delivery Systems

INPATIENT REHABILITATION

Recovery from injuries and illnesses is often made possible through **inpatient rehabilitation**. This process makes use of therapists and physicians who provide rehabilitation while the patient stays at a medical or rehabilitation hospital. Patients in inpatient rehabilitation either require intensive medical care, intensive therapy, or both. Rehabilitation may include a combination of physical, occupational, respiratory, cognitive, and speech therapy.

Patients in a medical hospital may receive therapy while they receive medical care. Typically, patients who require therapy and continued medical care will be moved to a **long-term acute care hospital (LTACH)**. In the hospital, medical needs will take priority, and the intensity of the therapy will depend on the patient's condition. Patients typically stay at an LTACH for ten to forty days before they are transferred to a lower level of care.

The most common diagnoses that require rehabilitation in a long-term acute care hospital are respiratory conditions (often involving a ventilator), including pulmonary edema, respiratory failure, pneumonia, and COPD. Other conditions that commonly require long-term hospitalization and rehabilitation include complex wounds (e.g., skin ulcers), septicemia, and degenerative musculoskeletal and connective tissue conditions.

Patients who are medically stable but require intensive therapy may be placed in an **inpatient rehabilitation hospital**. The patient will receive minimal medical care but will take part in several hours of therapy a day. The therapy is deemed necessary by a physician so that the patient can recover and safely return home.

Patients recovering from illness or injury in a **skilled nursing facility** will also be medically stable but will have less intense therapy sessions than those offered in an inpatient rehabilitation hospital. Skilled nursing facilities may focus on preparing patients to return home, but many also have the option to transfer patients to in-house long-term care communities.

PRACTICE QUESTION

1. Mrs. Jones is a fifty-year-old patient at a local hospital who is recovering from a stroke. She is medically stable and is not cognitively impaired. However, she will require physical therapy to regain gross and fine motor function. Where should Mrs. Jones start her rehabilitation?

   A) a long-term acute care hospital

   B) a skilled nursing facility

   C) an inpatient rehabilitation hospital

   D) her home

OUTPATIENT REHABILITATION

For people who do not require medical care and are able to live at home, rehabilitation may also be completed in an outpatient setting. The setting for outpatient rehabilitation will depend on the patient's needs and mobility.

Patients who do not need medical care but still need intense therapy often benefit from an outpatient **day program**, which provides daily therapy for several hours in a clinical setting. Patients have access to the specialized equipment they need and may work with a team of therapists from different fields.

Many hospitals and clinics offer **outpatient rehabilitation** for patients who may benefit from shorter therapy sessions (an hour or less per day). For example, a patient who is recovering from a heart procedure but no longer needs nursing care may want to improve his strength and endurance. Using a treadmill with the supervision of a physical therapist for thirty minutes a day may help him reach his health care goals.

Some patients cannot leave their home because of their health conditions, so they cannot attend therapy sessions in a clinical setting. These patients may be offered **home health rehabilitation** services per their physician's orders. In this case, the therapist comes to the patient's home. The frequency and duration of therapy sessions are determined by the patient's need and often by their insurance coverage.

For Medicare patients to be fully covered for home health rehabilitation, patients must be considered homebound. They do not have to be bedridden, but it must take a great deal of effort for them to leave their home. In addition, the therapy must be specialized, meaning the person could not perform the therapy on their own.

PRACTICE QUESTION

2. Which of these patients is considered eligible for Medicare-covered home health rehabilitation services?

    A) Lucy, who is recovering from alcoholism and works at the local grocery store

    B) George, who had a heart attack and is rebuilding cardiovascular endurance using a treadmill

    C) Peggy, a patient with Alzheimer's disease who recently fractured her hip

    D) Paul, an office manager who fractured his ankle on a camping trip

Functional Capacity Evaluation

The **Functional Capacity Evaluation (FCE)** is an exam that gauges someone's physical ability to do work-related tasks. It is performed by either a physician, physical therapist, or occupational therapist in a non-workplace setting. The client's treating physician cannot perform the FCE.

> Returning to the same job after an injury may not be realistic because of the extent of the injury. In this case, job modification or evaluation for an alternative job will be the focus of the FCE.

A variety of people may benefit from an FCE. Injured workers, whether they were injured on the job or injured outside of work, such as from a catastrophic accident, may need an FCE. These clients want to return to work. People who want to receive Social Security disability benefits may need to complete the evaluation to see whether they qualify. In addition, students who want to transition from school to work may benefit from an FCE.

To perform an FCE, a professional closely examines and documents the physical demands of a job. Job requirements may include pushing, pulling, sitting, standing, squatting, lifting, climbing stairs, or gripping items. The FCE will record any difficulty the client experiences doing the tasks and the time that each task takes.

PRACTICE QUESTION

3. Mercedes was injured at work, and she is ready to return to her former position. An FCE is requested. Who CANNOT perform the FCE?

    A) Mercedes's primary care physician

    B) an occupational therapist

    C) a physical therapist

    D) a physician in the community

Rehabilitation Strategies
Rehabilitation from Work-Related Injury

Workers' compensation may cover rehabilitation for a worker who was injured on the job. A **workers' compensation case manager** or **vocational case manager** is often hired to help the injured employee recover and return to work as soon as possible. This CCM can become involved during any point in the worker's recovery.

The CCM may provide telephonic duties such as triage immediately after an injury. The worker may not know whether the injury calls for a visit to the emergency department, and the worker may be seeking medical advice. The CCM will guide the worker to the appropriate medical setting if medical care is needed.

> If an injury or illness happens outside of work, workers' compensation benefits do not apply. These unfortunate clients may lose medical benefits as well as income if returning to work is not an option. The CCM should help these clients apply for Social Security Disability Insurance (SSDI) or Supplemental Security Income (SSI) or both.

The CCM may also assist with communication between the medical provider, client, employer, attorneys, and claims adjusters. Serving as the primary point of communication helps keep all parties on the same page during the injured worker's healing progress. As part of this process, the case manager will meet the injured worker and their family in the hospital, family home, or rehabilitation center to discuss care-plan goals and progress. Field CCMs will also attend meetings and medical appointments.

The case manager may also help determine the worker's ability to return to work and arrange the appropriate level of rehabilitation. The case manager must know the job requirements to determine what skills are needed to return the injured worker to the same job. To identify those requirements, the case manager will conduct a **functional job analysis (FJA)**, a study of the activities and responsibilities specific to that job. The case manager conducts the FJA by interviewing the worker and other employees and may also visit the job site. The FJA should include a description of all elements of the job, including:

+ responsibilities and performance standards
+ equipment used
+ work environment
+ scheduling requirements
+ body mechanics (e.g., standing or climbing)
+ relationship to other jobs in the company (e.g., does this job require supervision or supervise others)

After injured workers have recovered from their injury, they may need additional services to return to their job. The FJA can be used to identify the gap between the worker's current abilities and the requirements of his job. Several options are available to close this gap, including work hardening, work conditioning, work adjustment, and transitional work duty.

Work hardening is the most intense form of rehab designed to return a worker to a specific job. Working on-site or in a simulated work environment, the worker will perform job-specific tasks under the supervision of a physical or occupational therapist. For example, the worker may lift a fifteen-pound box and place it on a conveyor belt repeatedly to help build strength and endurance.

Work conditioning is typically less intensive than work hardening and does not focus on job-specific tasks. Instead, the focus is on rebuilding general strength, endurance, and/or mobility.

Work adjustment focuses on the social skills needed to succeed on the job, such as working with a team, being on time, and working under supervision. This work is often done in a group setting where workers can interact to simulate the interpersonal interactions common in a work setting. Work adjustment may be needed for employees who have traumatic brain injuries. For these employees, relearning effective communication and interpersonal skills is crucial.

 Work adjustment may be used to help clients learn appropriate hygiene, a skill that is important for returning to work.

Transitional work duty can be offered to employees who are able to work but in a different capacity. For example, a factory worker with a broken leg may be temporarily assigned to an office position within the company until their injury has healed. By using transitional work duty, workers are able to receive a steady paycheck and companies are able to use the skills and knowledge of trained workers. Transitional duty can be modified duty (a modified version of the original job) or an alternative position (an entirely different job).

Table 6.1. Vocational Rehabilitation

Type of Rehabilitation	Description
Work hardening	The employee goes through intense rehabilitation three to five days a week; this allows the employee to return to full employment.
Work conditioning	The employee goes through moderate rehabilitation two to four days a week; this focuses on rebuilding physical functioning so the employee can return to work.
Work adjustment	The employee goes through rehabilitation that focuses on behaviors that are important to success in the workplace.
Transitional work duty	The employee returns to work and performs job duties that have been modified to fit their capacity.

An injured worker reaches **medical maximum improvement (MMI)** when the medical provider determines that further rehabilitation would not improve the worker's condition. At this point, the case manager must help determine if the worker can return to their job, should move to a different job, or should plan on not returning to work. If returning to work is not an option for an injured worker, the CCM may help them access federal and state resources to provide long-term income. This income may include a settlement with the worker's employer and insurance company.

PRACTICE QUESTION

4. Ari was injured at work, and he lost the use of his right arm. He is doing rehabilitation to build strength and gain function of his injured arm. Which type of rehabilitation services is he most likely using?

    A) work conditioning

    B) work adjustment

    C) work hardening

    D) transitional work duty

REHABILITATION POST HOSPITALIZATION

After hospitalization for injury or illness, rehabilitation may be a part of the patient's post-hospitalization care plan. Case managers work with the patient, medical providers, and insurance providers to create a care plan specific to the patient's needs. Case managers help transfer patients from higher to lower levels of care as rehabilitation progresses and help the patient avoid rehospitalization.

The type and intensity of rehabilitation will depend on the injury or illness. For example, an employee who had a heart attack may need outpatient cardiac rehabilitation, while a patient recovering from a stroke may require a mix of physical, cognitive, and speech therapy in an inpatient setting. Providers who may be included in a post-hospitalization rehabilitation plan include cardiac, pulmonary, neurology, and addiction specialists. Psychiatrists and physical, occupational, and speech therapists may also play a role in such a plan.

> The **Functional Independence Measure (FIM) instrument** is used to assess patient motor and cognitive function during rehabilitation. Scores range from 1 (total dependence) to 7 (total independence). The **WeeFIM** assesses the same abilities in children using the same scale.

The CCM serves as an advocate for patients post-hospitalization, ensuring that they get the medical care they need. Coordination of care is a priority, and case managers may serve as a voice for their clients if necessary. The CCM may communicate with multiple medical providers to ensure the care is being provided as specified in the care plan and that the plan is up to date. The CCM will also communicate with insurance companies to ensure that services are being provided at the correct cost. The CCM may also help get medical equipment and research community resources that could help the patient.

5. Janice, a CCM, has a new client who had a massive stroke. He has lost significant motor and cognitive function. Which goal on the care plan created by Janice is reasonable and achievable?

   A) The client will drive to all medical appointments within two weeks of leaving the hospital.

   B) The client will discuss his emotional concerns with the psychiatrist within one week of beginning rehabilitation.

   C) The client will have resources in place for a wheelchair when he leaves the hospital.

   D) The client will begin physical therapy within two days of being admitted to the hospital for acute care.

Vocational Aspects of Chronic Illness and Disability

JOB ACCOMMODATIONS AND MODIFICATIONS

Work may be quite challenging for employees who are chronically ill or disabled. The CCM can help clients receive job accommodations so that people with disabilities can access employment and so that injured workers may return to work.

The Americans with Disabilities Act (ADA) requires employers to provide accommodations for workers with medical conditions. **Accommodations** are adjustments to the job, work environment, or hiring process that allow people with disabilities to fulfill the duties of a particular position. There are six categories of job accommodations that are listed in the ADA:

   ✦ assistive devices (e.g., computer braille display)

   ✦ building modification (e.g., ramps)

   ✦ job restructuring (e.g., shifting marginal tasks to another employee)

   ✦ job reassignment (e.g., assignment to a new position)

   ✦ personal assistant (e.g., a person to help the worker eat or use the restroom)

   ✦ training (e.g., learning how to perform a job duty)

It is the responsibility of the worker to request accommodations. The CCM can help the client get these accommodations. The case manager identifies the client's job-related limitations, identifies the relevant accommodations, and then works with the client and their employer to implement them.

Job modifications can make this task easier by changing the job description to suit the client's realistic capabilities. A job modification may require sharing job duties with a coworker, restructuring the job, or changing the company's policies.

> 🔍 The phrase *job modifications* is often used interchangeably with *job accommodations*. Sometimes it is used to refer specifically to changing the responsibilities of a job to meet the needs of employees with medical conditions.

Some accommodations can be made easily and cheaply by employers. For example, adjusting company policy to allow service animals or reassigning marginal tasks will have no cost for the employer. At other times, the job accommodations may be quite costly. Expanding a bathroom or hiring a personal assistant may require significant financial input from the company. Employers may reject accommodations if they create **undue hardship**, meaning they are too difficult or expensive to implement. Assisting clients with job accommodations may include negotiating with employers or helping clients submit claims to the **US Equal Employment Opportunity Commission (EEOC)** if the worker is being discriminated against.

PRACTICE QUESTION

6.   An employee with a disability needs a job accommodation to return to work. Which accommodation would NOT be awarded under the ADA?

   A)   building a wheelchair ramp

   B)   providing a stipend to cover medical expenses

   C)   bringing in a personal assistant to help with job duties

   D)   installing voice-recognition software on her computer

VOCATIONAL REHABILITATION

A person with a disability may be eligible for **vocational rehabilitation**, which is a federal program specialized to meet each person's specific employment needs. A vocational counselor will work one-on-one with the person to provide them with the skills, knowledge, and equipment needed to find realistic employment. People receiving Social Security Disability Insurance or Supplemental Security Income (or both) are eligible for vocational rehabilitation. However, if the person has a disability that is too severe to achieve employment, vocational rehabilitation may not be used.

Ticket to Work is a specific vocational rehabilitation program that is run out of state vocational rehabilitation agencies or through privately contracted **employment networks**. The program is available to people age eighteen to sixty-four who receive disability benefits from Social Security. Ticket to Work services include job training and placement, career counseling, and vocational rehabilitation. Clients who participate in the program should understand that its goal is to reduce or eliminate the need for Social Security benefits.

7. Which of the following individuals would be eligible to participate in the Ticket to Work program?

A) a factory worker who broke his arm on the job and will not be able to work for six weeks

B) a man with muscular dystrophy who receives Social Security Disability Insurance

C) a woman who receives Social Security Disability Insurance after a stroke left her homebound with significant cognitive impairments

D) an office worker with visual impairments who requires accommodations to perform her job duties

SUPPORTED EMPLOYMENT

People with significant disabilities may also become employed through federal **supported employment** programs, which help these people find, train for, and maintain employment. The setting for the work is an **integrated environment** alongside employees who do not have disabilities, and the work may be long term. The pay rate is competitive, and workers are matched to a job that uses their specific skills.

The case manager may help the person with a disability find rewarding, satisfying work. After completing an assessment, the case manager will have a broader knowledge of the client's skills and the skills that they may need to be taught. Learning about what type of work the client is looking for will guide the case manager's job search. Community businesses will be notified, and the hiring process will begin.

> Employees who have disabilities may work alongside employees who do not have disabilities in a supported employment environment. This situation creates workplace cohesion, and it allows the person with a disability to be a valuable part of the working community.

Clients who receive this service may have conditions that affect their concentration or information processing, such as schizophrenia, traumatic brain injuries, or personality disorders. Some may have sensory disabilities such as low vision, blindness, or being hard of hearing or deaf. Many clients will have lost limbs, and they will need specialized assistance. The case manager may help their clients acquire assistive-technology training and obtain assistive devices. The goal is to get the client into a job that may be long term and provide a higher quality of life.

Although funding and programs differ from state to state, federally funded vocational-rehabilitation agencies and county developmental-disability programs are commonly used. The case manager may work with the family to research all funding and community resources that are available for the client.

8.   Kiara provides case management services for supported employment. Which person
      would NOT qualify for Kiara's services?

      A)   Ahmed, who has been blind since birth

      B)   Michelle, who has just graduated from college without family or community
              assistance

      C)   John, whose personality disorder causes socialization problems in the workplace

      D)   Natalie, who lost both of her legs in a work-related accident

Assistive Devices

Assistive devices (or assistive technology) are pieces of equipment or technology that are
designed to help people with disabilities perform a task or an activity. They can be for home
use or may be available as job accommodations. There are many types of assistive devices that
vary from cheap and simple to expensive and complex. Assistive devices assist with specific
tasks, including:

+   mobility (e.g., wheelchairs, canes, prosthetic devices)

+   fine motor function (e.g., pencil grips, specialized handles, adaptive utensils)

+   hearing (e.g., hearing aids, closed captioning)

+   vision (e.g., magnifiers, screen readers)

+   communication (e.g., picture boards, voice output communication devices)

+   environmental access (e.g., ramps, automatic doors)

+   cognition and orientation (e.g., calendars, recording devices, location devices)

Funds for assistive devices can come from a variety of sources. Assistive devices needed
for work should be provided by the employer (unless they place an undue hardship on the
company). Vocational rehabilitation programs may also provide assistance acquiring assistive
devices. It can be more difficult for the case manager to find funds for assistive devices that are
needed for daily living. Some devices (durable medical equipment) are covered under Medicare,
and insurance providers may cover assistive devices that a physician deems medically necessary.
Also, private organizations, often associated with a particular condition, can help cover the cost
of assistive devices or can connect clients with donors or secondhand dealers.

PRACTICE QUESTION

9.   Which of the following is an assistive device most likely to be covered by Medicare?

      A)   crutches

      B)   zipper pulls

      C)   non-slip bath mat

      D)   screen reader

Answer Key

1. A) Incorrect. Mrs. Jones is medically stable and no longer needs medical care.

    B) Incorrect. She will require more intensive therapy than is offered in a skilled nursing facility and does not need the additional nursing care.

    C) Correct. She is medically stable and needs the intensive therapy offered at an inpatient rehabilitation hospital.

    D) Incorrect. Mrs. Jones does not yet have the motor function necessary to live at home.

2. A) Incorrect. Lucy works and is not homebound.

    B) Incorrect. George can use a treadmill without the services of a specialized therapist.

    C) Correct. Because of Peggy's disease and injury, it takes a great effort for her to leave her home.

    D) Incorrect. Although a fractured ankle may temporarily hinder Paul's mobility, he is not considered homebound.

3. **A) Correct.** The medical opinion needs to be unbiased, so her primary care physician cannot perform the FCE. The other answer choices are professionals who may perform the FCE.

4. **A) Correct.** Work conditioning focuses on restoring function.

    B) Incorrect. Work adjustment focuses on behavioral health issues.

    C) Incorrect. Work hardening is intense rehabilitation and likely beyond Ari's needs, given the scope of his injury.

    D) Incorrect. Transitional work duty provides lower-capacity work until the injury is healed.

5. A) Incorrect. The client will not drive so soon after leaving the hospital. He is likely to be transferred to a skilled nursing facility for rehabilitation.

    B) Incorrect. The client has had a brain injury, and processing information will likely still be difficult after one week of rehabilitation.

    C) Correct. Though the client will likely not need a wheelchair until he returns home, Janice should be preparing those resources before the client leaves the hospital.

    D) Incorrect. Two days is unreasonable to begin physical therapy after a massive stroke.

6. A) Incorrect. The Department of Labor acknowledges wheelchair ramps as a job accommodation.

    B) Correct. Under the ADA, an employer is not required to provide an extra stipend for medical expenses.

    C) Incorrect. Personal assistants would not cause undue hardship.

D)   Incorrect. A new computer program should not cause undue hardship to the employer.

7.   A.   Incorrect. Ticket to Work is not for people with temporary injuries who will return to work.

     B.   Correct. Ticket to Work is for people with disabilities who collect Social Security Disability Insurance and who are able to work.

     C.   Incorrect. A woman who is homebound and has significant cognitive impairments is unlikely to find work through Ticket to Work.

     D.   Incorrect. A person with disabilities who already has employment is not eligible for Ticket to Work.

8.   A)   Incorrect. Ahmed has a blindness disability, so he qualifies for supported employment.

     B)   Correct. Michelle has no disabilities, so she does not qualify for supported employment.

     C)   Incorrect. John has a personality disorder, so he qualifies for Kiara's services.

     D)   Incorrect. Natalie has a physical disability, so she qualifies for supported employment.

9.   **A)   Correct.** Crutches are durable medical equipment, which is covered by Medicare. The other items are not medical equipment and thus are not covered.

SEVEN: ETHICAL, LEGAL, AND PRACTICE STANDARDS

Health Care and Disability Related Legislation

AFFORDABLE CARE ACT

The **Affordable Care Act (ACA)** is a United States health reform federal statute signed into law by President Barack Obama on March 23, 2010. This landmark legislation aims to improve quality, affordability, and access in health care. To improve health care access, the ACA eliminated the denial of insurance coverage due to a pre-existing condition. Insurance companies also cannot charge more because of the condition or based on gender. Access to health care is improved by allowing adults who cannot obtain health insurance through a job to remain on their parents' policies until the age of twenty-six. Other components of the ACA improve affordability such as the closure of "the doughnut hole" for Medicare beneficiaries by 2020. This is a point in insurance coverage in which the beneficiary pays out of pocket for prescription drugs until a certain dollar amount is spent. Depending on the insured's age, free preventative care is also included as an insurance benefit.

The ACA must cover what are considered essential health benefits in the individual and small group insurance market. These benefits must be covered without annual dollar caps. There are ten health benefit categories:

+ Hospitalization
+ Mental health and substance abuse
+ Prescription drugs
+ Emergency treatment
+ Outpatient services
+ Maternity and care for the newborn
+ Rehabilitative and habilitative services and equipment
+ Laboratory services

+ Chronic disease management and preventative services
+ Pediatric services that include vision and oral care

Medicare restructures established by the ACA are intended to improve patient care while eliminating unnecessary health care costs. For example, one restructure provides financial incentives to hospitals and physicians that provide quality care. The hospital readmission reduction program allows Medicare to reduce payments to hospitals based on an excess readmission ratio process.

PRACTICE QUESTION

1. Which benefit listed below is NOT considered an essential health benefit under the ACA?

    A) behavioral health counseling

    B) adult dental

    C) prescriptions

    D) newborn care

AMERICANS WITH DISABILITIES ACT

The **Americans with Disabilities Act (ADA)** is a civil rights law that was established in 1990. The law prohibits discrimination against individuals who are determined to be disabled. This population deserves a quality of life equal to that enjoyed by individuals who do not have disabilities. Hence the ADA's purpose is to ensure the disabled population has equal rights in employment, transportation, schools, and all other public activities.

> The ADA states that an individual with a disability may be someone with a prior drug addiction. That person must not be currently using illegal drugs and may be randomly drug tested in certain circumstances.

The ADA defines disabilities in order to determine individuals who will be protected under the law. These individuals must have a mental or physical impairment that substantially limits one or more major life activities. The person may have a record or history of such impairments or is perceived by others, such as the employer, as having such limiting impairments.

The employer also has rights under the ADA. The disabled applicant must be able to perform the job and meet the same screening requirements, such as education, skills, or licenses. Persons with disabilities may require job **accommodations**, adjustments in the job duties or environment. Employers must provide these accommodations as long as they are reasonable and do not cause "undue hardship" to the employer, such as high expense or difficult installation.

Parts of Title I of the ADA outline reasonable accommodations. The job application process may need to be adjusted, for example. A blind or deaf person may need another person to attend the interview to assist with interpretation or literacy needs. Modifying the work environment is another area under Title I. For example, the employer may install a wheelchair ramp or provide a computer screen reader. Work schedules may also need modification.

The case manager may be of great assistance to the disabled worker. The case manager may need to research community services and set up transportation. The case manager may need to speak with the disabled client's employer and family to ensure all client needs are met for successful employment. The CCM will closely monitor a patient-centered care plan that includes achievable goals to help keep the client on track and ensure the client is content with their chosen job.

PRACTICE QUESTION

2. The ADA states that reasonable accommodations must be met for disabled employees. Which example accommodation listed below may NOT be awarded under the ADA?

   A) a new bathroom to accommodate an employee who uses a power wheelchair

   B) longer breaks for an employee who has type 1 diabetes

   C) a recorder that has frequent job task reminders for an employee with a developmental disability

   D) a basket and cushion for an employee with a physical disability

OCCUPATIONAL SAFETY AND HEALTH ADMINISTRATION

Employers are required to provide a safe workplace that is free from serious recognized hazards. This requirement is accomplished by setting and enforcing **Occupational Safety and Health Administration (OSHA)** standards. Congress created OSHA in the Occupational Safety and Health Act of 1970. OSHA is a component of the United States Department of Labor and covers private sector employers and their workers. OSHA provides education, assistance, outreach, and training to achieve its mission of safe working environments.

To support workplace safety, both employers and employees have responsibilities under OSHA standards. The employer must inspect the workplace for hazards and take the necessary steps to eliminate any hazards. The employer must also train employees to recognize safety and health concerns and take precautions to prevent accidents. If an accident or illness does occur, the employer must keep records according to OSHA's guidelines.

Employees must report any injury or illness and adhere to their employer's health and safety rules. If an OSHA officer inspects the organization, the employee must cooperate with the compliance officer. OSHA may inspect any workplace to ensure regulations are followed; however, search warrants may be required at times.

An occupational health nurse case manager coordinates comprehensive health care services following an employee injury or illness. The CM in this role will coordinate care to help the client return to work in the pre-illness or -injury state or with the highest level of functioning. The CM will assess, plan, implement, and evaluate to create actions required to achieve this goal.

PRACTICE QUESTION

3. OSHA sets standards to keep employees safe at work. Which of the following is NOT addressed by OSHA standards?

A) limiting exposure to hazardous chemicals

B) fall protection for workers who use ladders

C) drug testing during the interview process

D) preventing transmission of specific infectious diseases

HEALTH INSURANCE PORTABILITY AND ACCOUNTABILITY ACT

Congress passed the **Health Insurance Portability and Accountability Act (HIPAA)** in 1996. HIPAA allows workers to continue or transfer health coverage when they change or lose a job. The reduction of fraud and abuse is covered under Title II of HIPAA.

The handling of health care information is a major focus of HIPAA. The HIPAA Privacy Rule and the Security Rule, developed by the Department of Health and Human Services, protect the privacy and security of certain health care information. This **protected health information (PHI)** includes:

✦ demographic information (name, address, phone numbers, SSN, etc.)

✦ information included in the medical record

✦ payment history

The case manager must follow HIPAA privacy and security policies. PHI must be safeguarded, released, and disposed of in the manner described by HIPAA. The only personnel who should have access to clients' PHI are those who require that information for treatment or administrative purposes (e.g., billing, scheduling). When medical records are no longer needed (a length of time usually specified by state regulations), they must be destroyed so the information cannot be retrieved.

 HIPAA's Security Rule establishes rules pertaining to the transfer of electronic records. The Privacy Rule sets national standards for the protection of health care information.

PHI can only be released under specific circumstances. A **Privacy Rule Authorization form** must be signed by the client; this form allows the provider to release information to the parties included in the form. Clients may also authorize the provider to release their PHI to others, usually family members. PHI can be shared within the health care team only when it is considered relevant to treatment. In addition, PHI should not be shared with anyone not directly involved in the patient's care.

Case managers may also need to share PHI with outside government agencies. HIPAA specifies that the case manager must warn authorities if harm (e.g., exploitation or abuse) to the client is suspected. The case manager may report a birth, death, or disease to the appropriate agencies as specified by public health laws.

Annual HIPAA training is a component of most medical careers. This ensures that faxing, internet communications, and phone delivery of clients' health care records, including personal notes and billing, are properly handled.

PRACTICE QUESTION

4. Which of the following is most likely a violation of HIPAA?

    A) using a password to log onto a shared computer

    B) shredding medical records when they are expired

    C) accessing the medical record of a client's parents

    D) faxing the results of an ultrasound to a client's primary care provider

HEALTH INFORMATION TECHNOLOGY FOR ECONOMIC AND CLINICAL HEALTH ACT

The **Health Information Technology for Economic and Clinical Health Act (HITECH Act)** was written to encourage the use of electronic health records (EHRs) and related technology. The Centers for Medicare and Medicaid Services (CMS) awards eligible professionals with incentives for using EHRs. This incentive program is called **Meaningful Use**. The program was created to improve public health while maintaining privacy and security of health information. CMS has several objectives for using EHRs:

+ electronic exchanges of summary of care: An **exchange of summary of care** (also referred to as a discharge summary) refers to the movement of a patient from one setting to another. For example, the exchange of summary of care is used when a patient is discharged from a hospital to a home or skilled nursing facility.

+ reporting specific cases to specialized client registries: Specific cases must be reported to a specialized registry, except for cancer, which is reported to a cancer registry.

+ structured electronic transmission of laboratory test results: Laboratory test results incorporated into the patient's health record improves coordination of care and allows quicker and easier access.

+ use of electronic discharge prescriptions: Electronic discharge prescriptions improve efficiency by transmitting prescriptions quickly to the patient's pharmacy of choice.

> Prescriptions must be considered permissible for electronic prescribing. This refers to certain controlled substances restrictions.

5. A provider wishes to earn a Meaningful Use incentive. Which objective listed below BEST helps to eliminate gaps in care?

    A) reporting specific cases

    B) structured electronic transmission of laboratory test results

    C) use of electronic discharge prescriptions

    D) electronic exchanges of summary of care

FAMILY AND MEDICAL LEAVE ACT

Certain life changes may require an employee to be absent from work. The **Family and Medical Leave Act of 1993 (FMLA)** allows for certain workers to have up to twelve unpaid workweeks a year and return to their same job or a job that is equivalent to it.

Situations that fall under the FMLA include:

+ pregnancy, adoption, or foster child placement

+ personal serious health condition

+ caring for a family member (spouse, child, or parent) with an illness or injury

+ exigent circumstances related to family military deployment

 Many states have expanded the provisions of the FMLA to include smaller employers, other family members with illnesses, or specific illness/injuries.

Situations that DO NOT fall under the FMLA include:

+ short-term illness

+ routine medical care

+ caring for extended family, including grandparents, siblings, and in-laws

The FMLA is a federal law that covers all public employers and any private employers with fifty or more employees who have worked for at least twenty workweeks in the last year. Qualified employees must have worked for their covered employer for twelve months and worked at least 1,250 hours during those twelve months.

The entire twelve weeks of leave do not have to be taken consecutively. If desired, it may be taken in blocks and paid if the employee elects to use accrued paid time-off (PTO) benefits. The employer is allowed to require that any PTO benefits be used. If the employee's leave is unpaid, the employee will pay for medical insurance in the amount that is deducted from each paycheck.

HR benefits departments often hire case managers to assist with leaves of absence. These FMLA case managers need to know how to properly navigate time-off requests that fall under FMLA, including how to coordinate relevant information between employer, employee, and health care providers. Managing workers' compensation claims and providing customer service to employees may also be part of the FMLA case manager job description.

PRACTICE QUESTION

6. Which of the following clients, all employed by a company covered by the FMLA, will most likely NOT be eligible for FMLA?

    A) an employee with a mother-in-law who is beginning in-home hospice care

    B) an employee who has recently adopted a three-year-old child

    C) an employee who was unexpectedly left without child care after his military spouse was deployed

    D) an employee recently diagnosed with lung cancer

MENTAL HEALTH PARITY AND ADDICTION EQUALITY ACT

The **Mental Health Parity and Addiction Equity Act (MHPAEA)** was enacted in 2008 to fill in the gaps in the Mental Health Parity Act of 1996 (MHPA). The MHPA states that insurance plans that offer mental health care benefits must manage them as they manage medical/surgical benefits (i.e., the insurance company cannot place limits on mental health benefits that it does not place on medical/surgical benefits). The MHPAEA extended these protections to include substance use disorders and specified limitations on how insurance companies could cover mental health and substance use disorder benefits.

> Not every health insurance plan is required to offer mental health benefits under the MHPAEA. However, the ACA has greatly extended insurance plan coverage and lists mental health care as an Essential Health Benefit.

Care management services are also a benefit of many insurance plans that offer mental health care or substance abuse treatment. MHPAEA requires this benefit to be covered if warranted. Often these clients are homeless or in jeopardy of becoming homeless. The case manager will be the point of service and direct the client to shelter, work, and community resources. The case manager will provide support with medical treatment and assist the client with learning independent living skills.

PRACTICE QUESTION

7. Which of the following best describes the Mental Health Parity and Addiction Equality Act (MHPAEA)?

    A) The MHPAEA requires insurance companies to cover mental health benefits.

    B) The MHPAEA prevents insurance companies from imposing limits to mental health benefits.

    C) The MHPAEA requires insurance companies to use the same benefit structure for mental health and medical/surgical benefits.

    D) The MHPAEA prevents insurance companies from denying coverage to people with substance use disorders.

Legal and Regulatory Requirements

TORTS AND MALPRACTICE LAW

A **tort** is a wrongful civil act. Tort laws involve accidental or intentional harm to a person or property, which results from the wrongdoing of a person or persons. **Negligence** is a type of tort, defined as failure to offer an acceptable standard of care that is comparable and reasonable to what a competent medical assistant, nurse, or other health care worker would provide in a similar situation. There are four types of negligence.

1. **Nonfeasance** is a willful failure to act when required.
2. **Misfeasance** is the incorrect or improper performance of a lawful action.
3. **Malfeasance** is a willful and intentional action that causes harm.
4. **Malpractice** occurs when professionals fail to properly execute their duties.

Malpractice is a common type of tort lawsuit. For medical malpractice to occur, four things must occur: the patient-physician relationship was established (duty), the professional neglected to act or acted improperly (dereliction), a negative outcome occurred from an action or lack of an action (direct cause), and the patient sustained harm (damages).

PRACTICE QUESTION

8. Which of the following patient complaints could warrant a potential medical malpractice lawsuit?

    A) My doctor refused to order an MRI for me even though I requested one.

    B) My nurse had to stick me five times to draw a blood sample.

    C) My grandfather with dementia is not receiving meals in his nursing home.

    D) My doctor gave me a first round of antibiotics that didn't treat my infection.

END-OF-LIFE ISSUES

Advance directives are documents that state the patient's wishes for medical decisions used in the event he or she becomes incapable of making decisions. These documents must be signed by the patient, witnessed by state policy, and notarized by a legal notary.

Durable power of attorney is a type of advance directive that entitles a chosen person to act as a representative for medical and/or financial decisions. The trusted person chosen to make the medical decisions is called a health care surrogate or agent, depending on primary residency. This person will work with health care providers to ensure that medical treatment is performed in the manner designated by the incapacitated person. The financial appointed person is commonly called the agent or attorney-in-fact. This role continues any financial responsibilities in the event of mental incapacity. This may include paying bills, depositing checks, filing income taxes, or monitoring investments.

A **living will** is an advance directive document that explains which treatments the client would like in the event they are unable to express such at the time of illness. A living will (or similar document) may dictate the level of life-saving measures taken in certain circumstances.

- ✦ **Do not resuscitate (DNR)** typically indicates that no heroic measures should be taken to sustain the patient's life.

- ✦ **Do not intubate (DNI)** indicates that the patient does not wish to be intubated if the need presents.

- ✦ **Allow natural death (AND)** indicates that the patient does not want any intervention that may sustain life or prevent a natural progression to death.

 Advance directives may also address organ donation and specify which organs a patient is choosing to donate and/or specific recipients.

The federal **Patient Self Determination Act of 1989 (PSDA)** requires that patients under Medicare and Medicaid be provided with information concerning their rights to make health care decisions. This legislation is intended to improve the use of advance directives and increase the appropriateness of care while safeguarding the patient's decision-making rights. The PSDA encourages patients to decide about the extent of medical care they want early in the care process.

With the PSDA, the patient can choose which treatments and care activities they wish to accept or refuse. Also, this act requires that all health care organizations recognize the advance directive(s). Under the PSDA, the facility must explain to the patient their rights under state law, including the patients' rights to make medical care decisions, such as refusing or accepting treatment options. Additionally, the patient is entitled to receive information regarding their right to create an advance directive.

PRACTICE QUESTION

9.   Roy, a client, was in an auto accident and is in a coma. He had a durable power of attorney on file and lists his mother as his agent for medical and financial needs. Which action listed below will Roy's mother most likely be able to do as his agent?

   A)   make legal decision about Roy's will if he passes

   B)   pay Roy's car payment

   C)   let Roy's father be co-agent

   D)   make medical decisions that she desires

Ethics of Care Delivery and Professional Practice

Ethics are moral principles, values, and duties. Whereas laws are enforceable regulations set forth by the government, ethics are moral guidelines set forth and formally or informally enforced by peers, the community, and professional organizations. Ethics include norms and duties. **Norm** is short for "normal," which is a behavior or conduct that is valued and usually expected. **Duties** are commitments or obligations to act in an ethical and moral manner.

The case manager is first and foremost an advocate for her client and must allow **autonomy**, meaning she honors the client's right to make his own choices. This obligation can create conflict and ethical dilemmas, particularly when family and multiple providers are involved in the client's care. The case manager must always act on behalf of the client and communicate the client's wishes effectively.

Other ethical values that should be followed by case managers include:

+ **beneficence**: respecting the decisions the client has made and fostering a safe environment

+ **fidelity**: the duty of the case manager to be honest and trustworthy

+ **justice**: doing what is right and fair for the client

+ **nonmaleficence**: the focus on quality care and refraining from harming others

+ **veracity**: the act of telling the truth and not falsifying information

A **code of ethics** is a statement of the expected behaviors of its members. This code may also set standards and disciplinary actions for violations, including suspension, censure, fines, or expulsion. The Commission for Case Managers Certification (CCMC) has guidelines to assist the CCM when making ethical decisions. These guidelines are referred to as the Code of Professional Conduct. If a CCM has an ethical concern, she is encouraged to contact the CCMC for advice.

PRACTICE QUESTION

10.   Which example below BEST describes beneficence?

   A)   allowing a patient to die as requested in her living will

   B)   explaining a surgical procedure to a nervous client

   C)   going to court with a client who is suing a health care provider

   D)   establishing boundaries with new clients

Guidelines, Standards, and Pathways

Patient care should follow guidelines, standards, and pathways built on evidence-based practice. Medical professionals research and develop **guidelines** to serve as flexible recommendations for quality care. Unlike guidelines, **standards of care** are not flexible: they are a set means to providing quality patient care.

Clinical pathways (also known as care pathways or care maps) are outcome-focused tools used by the medical team to care for a group of patients receiving the same type of interventions. This tool or algorithm is typically a bedside document that defines the care needed to return the patient to optimum health. Each step is sequential and includes specific outcomes. Clinical pathways may include detailed instructions for treatment, medication, observation, diagnostics, nutrition, mobility, and education.

Standards of practice are statements of expected professional behavior and care developed by professional organizations. The **Commission for Case Manager Certification (CCMC)** is a nationally accredited organization that certifies case managers. The CCMC's Code of Professional Conduct defines a set of standards, rules, procedures, and penalties for case managers. The CCMC's primary objective is to protect the public interest. The standards of practice are outlined in multiple sections. Topics covered are:

+ the client advocate

+ professional responsibility

+ case manager/client relationships

+ confidentiality, privacy, security, and recordkeeping

+ professional relationships

Case managers with other licenses must follow the standards of practice set by those organizations. For example, an RN must follow standards of practice set by the American Nursing Association (ANA).

The **Case Manager Society of America (CMSA)** is a case management membership organization that is an approved provider of continuing education to maintain certification with CCMC. CMSA recognizes standards of practice guidelines that are essential to identify and address the knowledge, skills, and competencies to be a successful case manager in a wide variety of settings.

PRACTICE QUESTION

11. Which of the following would most likely be a violation of the CCM standards of practice?

A) A CCM does not impose her values on her client.

B) A CCM transfers her credentials to an organization.

C) A CCM works with her client to develop goals.

D) A CCM keeps client records protected.

Case Recording and Documentation

The case manager is responsible for maintaining accurate, objective documentation of the client's care. Accurate documentation has obvious benefits for the patient's care but is also important for the CCM. CCMs can use accurate, timely documentation to prove they have complied with standards of care and practice, which is important both for professional advancement and for a possible legal defense.

Because case managers work in a variety of health care environments, documentation will rely on the setting. The role of the case manager and the standards maintained by her employer will dictate the format and information included in the client's record. However, there are several general guidelines CMs should follow.

+ Only document facts; the case worker's opinions do not belong in official documentation.

+ Record details of the client visit as soon as possible after the visit.

+ Always record if the client agrees or refuses case management, interventions, or other types of care.

+ Record all communication with people or organizations involved in the client's care, including the client's family, medical providers, employer, and insurance companies.

+ Document the care plan, including assessments, interventions, evaluations, and the outcomes.

+ Document modifications of the care plan and the rationale for the changes.

+ Include all legal documents, including advance directives and consent forms.

+ Document discharge plans and patient education.

PRACTICE QUESTION

12.   What is the best rationale for why timely documentation is so important for the case manager?

   A)   to establish a rapport with the client

   B)   to ensure advance directives are enforced

   C)   to defend against a claim of negligence

   D)   to begin educating the client and family

Risk Management

Caring for patients always comes with risk to both the patient and the health care provider. **Risk management** is a process designed to help reduce adverse events and make corrections after adverse events have occurred. In some settings, case managers will act as risk managers to identify potential risks or determine the probability of an adverse event. Because financial loss is a part of adverse events, the CM may also need to estimate the costs associated with a specific adverse event.

When an adverse event has occurred, reactive risk management is employed. A common tool used for this type of risk management is the **root cause analysis (RCA)**. The RCA does not blame individuals for their errors; it centers on system mistakes. There are specific steps to be taken within the RCA.

1.   Data is collected and interpreted to reconstruct the event.

2.   A multidisciplinary team analyzes the data using causal factor charting.

3. The root cause (error(s) that caused the event) is identified.

4. A plan is formulated to prevent future adverse events.

PRACTICE QUESTION

13. A nurse accidentally gave a patient a double dosage of a medication. Risk management is involved to identify the potential for reoccurrence. Which example below should be the primary focus of the RCA?

    A) determining why the nurse made the error

    B) calculating financial losses

    C) determining the medication system used by the nurse

    D) decreasing malpractice claims

Self-Care and Well-Being as a Professional

Being a case manager can be a challenging, stressful job. CCMs will often have clients who are dealing with illness, death, or financial hardship, and the emotional work of managing these clients can be immense. Case managers will also have to navigate complex systems, such as hospitals, insurance companies, and government agencies.

Because of these strains, the CCM should not overlook his own self-care. The CCM cannot serve his client well if he is not taking good care of himself. There are many ways the CCM may fulfill the goal of being healthy and happy. Routine exercise and eating a well-balanced diet will improve health and provide energy. Getting adequate sleep, enjoying hobbies, and relaxing and spending time with friends and family also improve self-care and well-being. The CCM should also set careful boundaries, both physical and emotional, with clients and be willing to ask for assistance when confronted with unmanageable tasks.

PRACTICE QUESTION

14. Which of the following is NOT an appropriate method of case manager self-care?

    A) keeping separate phones for professional and private contacts

    B) refusing to answer calls from a client who is verbally abusive

    C) setting aside an hour a day to eat lunch and take a walk

    D) contacting the CCMC when struggling with an ethical dilemma presented by a client

Answer Key

1. **B)** **Correct.** Pediatric dental is included, but adult dental care is not. The other choices are essential health benefits under the ACA.

2. **A)** **Correct.** Constructing a new bathroom may cause undue hardship to the employer as it could be both expensive and disruptive to the company's work.
   B) Incorrect. Work schedules may be modified under the ADA.
   C) Incorrect. A tape recorder would not be a costly accommodation.
   D) Incorrect. A cushion and a basket are reasonable, inexpensive accommodations.

3. **C)** **Correct.** OSHA may drug test persons involved in workplace accidents, but the agency does not set standards for drug tests that occur during the hiring process. OSHA sets standards for the situations described in the other choices.

4. A) Incorrect. Passwords are vital for electronic records and should be used on every computer in the medical office.
   B) Incorrect. Records containing PHI have expiration dates and need to be shredded at that time.
   C) **Correct.** Under HIPAA, the case manager is not allowed to access the medical records of people whose care she is not involved in.
   D) Incorrect. Faxing test results should fall under the Privacy Rule Authorization form signed by the client at the beginning of their care.

5. A) Incorrect. Reporting specific cases to registries helps with identification of specific cases and trends.
   B) Incorrect. Structured electronic transmission of laboratory test results improves access to those results, but exchanges of summary of care provide more information for better coordination of care.
   C) Incorrect. Electronic discharge prescriptions ensure that medications are prescribed quickly.
   D) **Correct.** Electronic exchanges of summary of care improve coordination of care.

6. **A)** **Correct.** The FMLA does not cover leave for employees to care for in-laws.
   B) Incorrect. The FMLA covers leave for all new parents following an adoption, pregnancy, or foster care placement.
   C) Incorrect. Leave for exigent circumstances caused by military deployment falls under the FMLA.
   D) Incorrect. This employee has a serious health condition that will likely require hospitalization or continual care, so they will likely qualify for FMLA.

7.
A) Incorrect. The ACA, not the MHPAEA, requires companies to cover mental health benefits.

B) Incorrect. The MHPAEA does not prevent companies from imposing limits on mental health benefits.

C) Correct. The MHPAEA requires that insurance companies not impose limits on mental health benefits that are different from the limits on medical/surgical benefits.

D) Incorrect. The MHPAEA does not dictate who can receive insurance coverage.

8.
A) Incorrect. The doctor is working within professional standards to deny an unnecessary MRI, even if the patient requests it.

B) Incorrect. While the nurse may not have met the required standard of care, the blood draw did not cause significant harm.

C) Correct. This patient may not be able to feed himself. A malpractice suit is warranted if the patient becomes malnourished and suffers related illness or injury.

D) Incorrect. The doctor has not violated standards of care: it is not unusual for the first round of antibiotics to be ineffective.

9.
A) Incorrect. She may not be the executor of Roy's will.

B) Correct. As financial agent, she may pay Roy's bills.

C) Incorrect. Unless Roy has specified his father as co-agent, he cannot be co-agent.

D) Incorrect. To the best of her ability, Roy's mother must make the medical decisions that he would desire.

10.
A) Correct. The CCM is allowing the client's wishes to be fulfilled.

B) Incorrect. The CCM is practicing veracity.

C) Incorrect. The CCM is practicing justice.

D) Incorrect. The CCM is practicing fidelity.

11.
B) Correct. A CCM may not transfer her credentials. The other choices are part of the CCM standards of practice.

12.
A) Incorrect. The rapport can be established without timely documentation.

B) Incorrect. Advance directives are separate from timely documentation.

C) Correct. Timely documentation may serve to defend the case manager.

D) Incorrect. Documentation should be timely with education, but this is not the best answer.

13.
A) Incorrect. Although it is important to discover why the nurse made the error, the RCA does not focus on human error.

B) Incorrect. Calculating financial losses is a component of the RCA but not the primary focus.

C) Correct. The RCA will focus on the medication system.

D) Incorrect. Decreasing malpractice claims is not the primary focus of the RCA.

14. A) Incorrect. Keeping separate professional and private phones is an appropriate way to set boundaries.

B) Correct. The CCM should not stop communicating with the client. Instead, the CCM should work with her supervisor and the client to manage the behavior in a way that minimizes the negative impact on the client's care.

C) Incorrect. A healthy diet and exercise are important components of self-care.

D) Incorrect. Reaching out to the CCMC with professional questions is an appropriate way to handle the stress of an ethical dilemma.

EIGHT: Practice Test

READ THE QUESTION, AND THEN CHOOSE THE MOST CORRECT ANSWER.

1. Disability case managers are most often employed by:

   A) the Social Security Administration.

   B) workers' compensation insurers.

   C) skilled nursing facilities.

   D) assisted living facilities.

2. The federal agency charged with improving the safety and quality of the United States health care system is:

   A) the Institute of Medicine (IOM).

   B) Health and Human Services (HHS).

   C) the Joint Commission.

   D) the Agency for Healthcare Research and Quality (AHRQ).

3. Colorectal cancer screening is recommended for:

   A) women of average risk at forty-five.

   B) men and women of average risk at forty-five.

   C) men and women of average risk at fifty.

   D) men and women of average risk at forty.

4. Case recording and good documentation are NOT meant to:

   A) justify expenses.

   B) defend the CCM against negligence.

   C) assist the family and friends in knowing the activities of the client.

   D) validate interventions.

5. The Functional Independence Measure (FIM) is a tool used by health care professionals. If the patient had a score of 7 on a scale, the evaluator would document that the patient:

   A) needed no assistance and was completely independent.

   B) needed minimal assistance with activities of daily living.

   C) needed total assistance with most activities.

   D) needed assistance with ambulation.

6. Part D of Medicare is also known as the:

   A) Medicare Supplemental Plan.

   B) Medicare Hospital and Long-Term Care Coverage.

   C) Medicare Prescription Drug Plan.

   D) Medicare Prescription Drug Advantage.

7. The CCM has a hospitalized patient who practices Hinduism and is refusing a common medical intervention. The CCM realizes this refusal may be related to any of the following Hindu beliefs EXCEPT:

   A) suffering being caused by past life experience.

   B) being prohibited from using Western medicine.

   C) the experience of pain promoting spiritual growth.

   D) the need for proper food prior to the treatment.

8. Your new client at a community health center has uncontrolled type 1 diabetes and nephropathy. He states that he can't get "disability" because he has never worked. You know he may be able to get SSI benefits because:

   A) he is over age fifty, so he qualifies for SSI.

   B) his parents worked, so he can collect on their benefits.

   C) SSI is for disabled people who may have never worked.

   D) SSI is administered by the state and covers disabled people.

9. Understanding the family dynamics when accepting a new patient is critical. In analyzing family dynamics, the CCM should seek to understand all of the following EXCEPT:

   A) knowing the patient's role in the family dynamics.

   B) knowing which family member is the main caregiver.

   C) modifications of family responsibilities due to the diagnosis.

   D) disease management services.

10. When determining the patient's role in family dynamics, the CCM should consider all of the following information EXCEPT:

    A) What type of career did the patient have, and were they the primary breadwinner?

    B) Did the patient ever care for anyone in the family?

    C) What medications does the patient take?

    D) Did the patient marry and have children?

11. To meet SSI income requirements, you can only have _____ in assets as an individual.

    A) $1,500

    B) $2,000

    C) $2,500

    D) $3,000

12. As a case management director at a large urban community health center, you are asked to prepare a presentation summarizing disparities in health care for the vulnerable populations that you serve. One data source you utilize to obtain information is the:

A) ORYX report.

B) CMS Patient Quality and Disparities Index.

C) National Healthcare Quality and Disparities Report.

D) CMS Health and Safety Report.

13. The vaccine that is NOT recommended for people born before 1957 is the:

A) herpes zoster.

B) influenza (flu shot).

C) pneumococcal (pneumonia).

D) measles, mumps, and rubella (MMR).

14. A recommended wellness strategy is:

A) thirty minutes of moderate physical activity a day.

B) thirty minutes of moderate activity three times per week.

C) shingles vaccine for adults over fifty.

D) annual colorectal screenings.

15. The four components of communication do NOT include:

A) the message.

B) the sender.

C) the format.

D) the context.

16. The CCM has different spiritual beliefs than their patient. An effective intervention for the patient would be to:

A) keep the CCM's beliefs separate from their patient care duties and ensure that the patient's beliefs are the only ones to impact their medical care.

B) encourage more pastoral visits for the patient.

C) provide the patient with education on the CCM's spiritual beliefs.

D) encourage more physician visits.

17. An example of inappropriate documentation is:

A) The patient ate 100 percent of their meal at 8:00.

B) The patient's outfit is not attractive; therefore, the patient didn't attend the outing.

C) The patient did not attend the outing due to reported feelings of depression.

D) The patient stated, "I feel depressed and do not want to go to the outing."

18. The Functional Independence Measure (FIM) is a tool that evaluates tasks to determine level of disability. This measure does NOT evaluate:

A) how the patient transfers.

B) how the patient communicates.

C) the social cognition of the patient.

D) how well the patient sleeps.

19. Social Security Disability Insurance (SSDI) is funded by:

A) the US Treasury Department.

B) a private disability reinsurer.

C) employers.

D) taxpayers.

20. A workers' compensation case manager is charged with creating a "physician report card" that will measure physician performance. One variable of this report card should be:

A) the number of clients who obtain Social Security Disability Insurance.

B) aggregate days of disability of all clients treated.

C) the usability of narrative reports.

D) mean days of disability per diagnosis.

21. According to the American Cancer Society, women should have a mammogram:

A) every other year after forty.

B) every year after forty.

C) every year between forty-five and fifty-four.

D) every year after fifty.

22. Which statement about documentation is incorrect?

A) Documentation with the family must be included.

B) Communication with the insurer must not be included.

C) Documentation should be done shortly after the encounter, if possible.

D) Rationale to modify the care plan should be documented.

23. Interpersonal communication is paramount for the CCM. Interpersonal communication does NOT include:

A) active listening.

B) nodding.

C) formulating necessary changes.

D) taking notes.

24. A family member of the patient calls the CCM to report a concern, but the CCM cannot hear them due to construction noise in the background. The construction noise is an example of this communication barrier:

A) physiological noise

B) structural barrier

C) physical interference

D) perceptual barrier

25. All of the following statements about the Inpatient Rehabilitation Facility–Patient Assessment Instrument (IRF–PAI) are true EXCEPT:

A) It is used for Medicare Part C patients.

B) It is used for Medicare Part A fee-for-service patients.

C) It is used to determine payment.

D) It is used solely for Medicaid patients.

26. Social Security Disability Insurance (SSDI) is for people who have sufficient work quarters and:

A) have a disability that prevents basic, substantially gainful work activities for at least one year.

B) have a disability and are over age fifty and can no longer work.

C) have a disability that is on the SSDI Listing of Impairments.

D) have a disability that prevents basic, substantially gainful work activities for at least three years.

27. A non-disabled person qualifies for Medicare at age:

A) sixty-seven.

B) sixty-six.

C) sixty-five.

D) sixty-four.

28. Health risks and outcomes for clients can be evaluated by using:

   A) a health assessment screening tool.

   B) a scan of past medical records.

   C) evidence-based guidelines.

   D) local hospital data.

29. The wellness goal that a CCM does NOT discuss with a patient unless recommended by a physician is:

   A) a routine foot exam for patients with diabetes.

   B) an annual flu vaccine.

   C) an annual audiology exam.

   D) an annual Medicare wellness exam.

30. A CCM observes a caregiver verbally abusing their patient. An inappropriate intervention by the CCM would be to:

   A) determine the reason the caregiver gets upset and help find appropriate support.

   B) report the abuse to elder protective services.

   C) call the police if immediate danger is suspected.

   D) ensure the safety of the patient and tell the caregiver that their anger is justified.

31. Medicare Part B provides coverage for:

   A) occupational therapy.

   B) outpatient hospital care.

   C) at-home hospice care.

   D) prescription drugs.

32. A patient of East Indian origin who is over sixty-five may receive _____ while hospitalized.

   A) personal attention from nurses

   B) pastoral visits

   C) family involvement in health care decisions

   D) privacy and confidentiality

33. The CCM works in a hospital setting. Potential documentation for a patient may include all of the following EXCEPT:

   A) informed consent.

   B) discharge planning.

   C) advance directives.

   D) outcome of physical therapy completion.

34. An own-occupation policy is NOT:

   A) a type of full disability insurance.

   B) the strictest type of disability policy.

   C) the most lenient type of disability policy.

   D) a high-cost policy.

35. A person who has been deemed eligible for SSDI will receive Medicare benefits:

   A) immediately.

   B) after one year.

   C) after two years.

   D) after three months.

36. Compared with urban residents, rural residents are:

   A) healthier and weigh less.

   B) poorer, older, and sicker.

   C) more prone to diabetes.

   D) happier and more self-directed.

37. The CCM has a new patient whose cultural practices conflict with his physician's treatment recommendations. The CCM realizes these practices may cause a health risk to the patient. After the patient is educated by the CCM, the final decision on the appropriate treatment plan will be made by:

A) the physician.

B) the patient.

C) the CCM.

D) the family.

38. The patient should expect that their treatment conforms to:

A) standards of care.

B) standards of practice.

C) clinical pathway.

D) practice guidelines.

39. When coordinating a transition of a client to another care provider, the case manager should always be aware that:

A) the client may not accept the transition.

B) the client is at increased risk for an adverse outcome.

C) the client is now the responsibility of the receiving provider.

D) the client's family must agree to the transition plan.

40. The state-federal program that provides health insurance for children is known as:

A) CIP.

B) CMMS.

C) NCLB.

D) CHIP.

41. A measure of a transition of care might include:

A) hospitalized COPD patients who were provided with complete discharge instructions.

B) patients who were discharged on time.

C) supplies that were given to indigent patients.

D) hospitalized diabetic patients who were satisfied with hospital services.

42. A provider being paid a capitated rate:

A) receives a predetermined global fee annually for participation in a plan.

B) is always a provider in a managed care organization (MCO).

C) receives a fee that is determined by CMS.

D) receives a predetermined fee for each patient in a plan.

43. A CCM disagrees with their patient's cultural beliefs regarding health care choices. It is the CCM's responsibility to:

A) educate the patient regarding their health needs and support the patient's beliefs even if the CCM disagrees.

B) educate and persuade the patient to comply with the correct intervention.

C) have a conference with the IDT and explore ways to persuade the patient to make the correct decision.

D) educate the family about the correct decision and see if they can persuade the patient.

44. The set of principles that states what is expected of a provider are:

A) standards of care.

B) standards of practice.

C) clinical pathway.

D) practice guidelines.

45. A long-term disability policy that strictly defines disability and is less expensive than some other policies is known as:

A) own-occupation.

B) any-occupation.

C) only-occupation.

D) long-term occupation.

46. Since the advent of the opioid crisis, many states have operationalized:

A) mandatory jail terms for abusive prescribers.

B) prescription drug monitoring programs.

C) forty-eight-hour holds on narcotic medications.

D) limitations on narcotic medication refills.

47. Off-label medication is:

A) made by a non-US pharmaceutical company and is not FDA approved.

B) purchased by illegal means.

C) prescribed for someone else.

D) prescribed for a purpose not specified by the FDA.

48. A significant contributor to rising health care costs is:

A) higher charges by specialists.

B) sicker patients.

C) readmissions.

D) Medicare fraud.

49. The CCM's new patient is a practicing Jehovah's Witness. The CCM understands that an important component of this religion that may affect the patient's medical decision is the belief that:

A) mental illness does not require medication.

B) preventive medical treatment is not important.

C) blood transfusions are not allowed.

D) medications are stopped once the symptoms of illness have ceased.

50. Standards of care are NOT:

A) strict and meant to be followed.

B) designed to be flexible.

C) medically necessary.

D) based on current outcomes data.

51. Trust is built with the patient through:

A) canceling and rescheduling appointments.

B) speaking over the patient to demonstrate knowledge.

C) doing what you say you will do.

D) doing what the patient wants.

52. The CCM is interviewing a new patient who frequently deviates from the questions. A good way for the CCM to redirect the interview is to:

A) use guided questions.

B) speak more quickly.

C) omit less important assessment questions.

D) inform the patient that only pertinent information is needed.

53. What is NOT true of home health rehabilitation?

A) The patient should not leave home, except for medical or short nonmedical trips.

B) Visits are typically four to five times per week.

C) Physical therapy is provided in the patient's home for an hour per session.

D) The patient no longer needs hospitalization but does need intensive therapy.

54. An effective way for the CCM to close the interview would be to:

A) request to meet with the family.

B) request a face-to-face visit.

C) explain the care plan.

D) ask to call the primary care physician.

55. A CCM's new patient has recently been diagnosed with insulin-dependent diabetes. The factor that will help the family adapt to the diagnosis is:

A) denying the condition of the patient.

B) relying on one family member for all duties.

C) researching and accepting help.

D) focusing on the patient and not the other family members.

56. An example of soft savings in case management practice would be:

A) a negotiated lower rate for DME.

B) hiring a medical assistant to provide case management.

C) precertification.

D) avoided emergency department (ED) visits.

57. The program that provides block grants to states to provide financial assistance and support to families is the:

A) Transitional Assistance to New Families.

B) Social Security Administration.

C) Temporary Assistance for Needy Families.

D) US Public Welfare Division.

58. A CCM is working in a hospital with a patient who is Jewish. The CCM understands that part of this religion may include:

A) following certain dietary guidelines.

B) limiting physical activity on certain days of the week.

C) avoiding eye contact in interpersonal interactions.

D) believing illness is caused by a disturbance in chi (energy).

59. Practice guidelines are NOT:

A) strict and meant to be followed.

B) designed to be flexible.

C) clinical recommendations.

D) meant to replace the provider judgments.

60. There are many barriers to effective communication. Barriers referred to as a prejudice of the listener include:

A) barrier to processing information.

B) perceptual filters.

C) physical interference.

D) semantic noise.

61. A medical home is a philosophy and model of primary care that is:

   A) patient centered.

   B) hospital affiliated.

   C) a telehealth system.

   D) part of a preferred provider network.

62. Susan works for a large health care insurance company as a case manager. She works with network physicians to provide optimal quality care for the plan members. This type of case management is also known as:

   A) payer-based case management.

   B) third-party case management.

   C) workers' compensation case management.

   D) primary care case management.

63. A cultural group whose beliefs include faith that certain foods may help heal illnesses is:

   A) followers of Judaism.

   B) practitioners of Traditional Chinese Medicine.

   C) practicing Jehovah's Witnesses.

   D) Christian Scientists.

64. Which item listed below is NOT typically a goal of the motivational interview process?

   A) evaluating the patient's care needs

   B) reinforcing the patient's statements regarding change

   C) discovering what concerns the patient about changing their behavior

   D) addressing the patient's care needs as a partnership

65. A review of services to determine medical necessity is known as:

   A) preadmission certification.

   B) utilization management.

   C) prequalification.

   D) quality assurance.

66. An important benchmark in workers' compensation case management is:

   A) reducing injuries.

   B) improving return-to-work times.

   C) managing caseloads.

   D) improving UR performance.

67. TRICARE allows military personnel to receive care:

   A) at the VA hospital system.

   B) at the VA hospital system or through private facilities.

   C) at predetermined facilities.

   D) when they are on active duty.

68. An Islamic belief that could conflict with medical recommendations regarding diabetes care may include:

   A) following a halal diet.

   B) fasting during Ramadan.

   C) prohibitions against injections.

   D) praying five times daily.

69. Algorithms that incorporate protocols for common diseases and procedures are called:

   A) evidence-based guidelines.

   B) clinical pathways.

   C) standards of practice.

   D) practice guidelines.

70. Older Chinese patients are likely to believe all of the following in relation to health care EXCEPT:

A) Avoiding eye contact with the MD is a sign of respect.

B) Illness may be caused by a disturbance in their chi (energy).

C) The head of the household is frequently involved in health care decisions.

D) Nodding in response to an authority figure is a sign of disrespect.

71. Your client, who was recently discharged from a skilled nursing facility, has had increasing issues with aspirating while eating. You would like the client's ability to swallow evaluated and recommend a referral to:

A) a speech pathologist.

B) a radiologist.

C) a dietician.

D) a respiratory therapist.

72. During a functional job analysis:

A) information is collected to define the patient's job duties.

B) interviews are performed with coworkers and supervisors.

C) job scheduling is not a concern.

D) a physical or occupational therapist may perform the analysis.

73. A primary benefit of having a spiritual practice is:

A) a more successful career.

B) more social engagements.

C) a longer life.

D) meeting familial expectations.

74. Important psychosocial resources for the CCM's patient would include:

A) transportation to medical appointments.

B) support groups.

C) wellness exams.

D) community events.

75. A network of providers and hospitals who agree to provide services to members for a lower reimbursement rate and with more freedom to select providers without a referral is known as a:

A) health management organization (HMO).

B) preferred provider organization (PPO).

C) hospital-centered network.

D) provider hospital network.

76. The longer an injured worker is out of work:

A) the more case management is needed.

B) the more likely she is to return to work in a new career.

C) the less likely she will ever return to work.

D) the less the claim costs over time.

77. The nonprofit group that collects data to evaluate the safety and quality performance of hospitals and provides that information to consumers is:

A) The American Medical Association.

B) The Leapfrog Group.

C) The Abacus Group.

D) Health and Human Services.

78. The implementation phase of a case management plan is also called:

A) an action plan.

B) objective attainment.

C) care coordination.

D) plan completion.

79. Evidence-based practice refers to:

A) using medical interventions that are proven through research to be effective.

B) recommendations for health and wellness goals.

C) rigid criteria to meet medical necessity requirements.

D) systemically developing statements that serve providers in determining care.

80. Patient autonomy does NOT:

A) focus on defending individuals who cannot represent themselves.

B) refer to patients having control over their own health care decisions.

C) describe a patient's freedom to make choices.

D) foster patient independence.

81. A rehabilitation CCM is seeing a new patient who was injured while driving his taxi. He cannot drive currently but can work in the office for the taxi company until he has healed from his injury. The CCM knows this situation is called:

A) Transitional Work Duty (TWD).

B) Work Adjustment.

C) Work Conditioning.

D) Job Development.

82. The cost of health insurance each month is known as the:

A) co-insurance.

B) co-pay.

C) premium.

D) deductible.

83. A CCM makes a house call to a fifty-year-old client with diabetes who has just returned home from a hospital stay. During the visit, the case manager observes his client's elderly mother lying on a urine-soaked bed. The client admits that no one was caring for his mother while he was in the hospital and states that a family member is going to come to help. As a result, the CCM should:

A) take care of the client's mother while at the home.

B) find out if the mother is eligible for in-home services.

C) report the situation to his supervisor.

D) report the situation to the appropriate state agency.

84. The regulatory body that performs accreditation of health systems and establishes national standards for quality measures is:

A) Health and Human Services.

B) The Leapfrog Group.

C) The Joint Commission.

D) The Hospital Quality Commission.

85. The best way for the CCM to begin an interview is by:

A) asking family members to attend.

B) asking open-ended questions.

C) asking that the patient be alone in a safe location.

D) asking for medication and health history lists.

86. Preparing for the patient interview is an important step for the CCM. This phase includes all of the following EXCEPT:

A) scheduling the interview when there will be no interruptions.

B) informing the patient about information that will be needed.

C) informing the patient of the interview's approximate duration.

D) creating goals for the patient's health needs.

87. Michael works in a community health clinic that focuses on vulnerable populations with insulin-dependent diabetes. He provides education, monitoring, and supplies for eligible clients. This type of case management is called:

A) community health case management.

B) public health case management.

C) diagnosis management.

D) disease management.

88. In patient care, beneficence is NOT:

A) an obligation to do good for the patient.

B) providing informed consent.

C) defined as the act of telling the truth.

D) removing the patient from harm's way.

89. Ergonomic products address:

A) renumeration and benefits.

B) environment and productivity.

C) legal and moral issues.

D) organization and cooperation.

90. Cultural competence in health care is best described as:

A) providing health care professionals that speak the patient's native language.

B) the integration of multicultural providers within a network.

C) the integration of a variety of factors such as race, ethnicity, language, and socioeconomic status into care delivery.

D) the ability to empathize with patients from a variety of cultures.

91. As a case manager in an inpatient detoxification facility, you are working to prepare a client for transfer to a residential treatment center. This activity is also known as:

A) discharge planning.

B) transitional discharge.

C) transition of care.

D) transfer care.

92. _____ serve designated high-need areas or populations.

A) Free clinics

B) Community-based centers

C) Medical homes

D) Community health centers

93. One of the most important outcome measures used by CMS to evaluate hospitals is:

A) cost of hospital stay.

B) mortality.

C) efficient use of medical imaging.

D) use of case management at discharge.

94. To improve an outcome, the _____ must be improved.

   A) process

   B) measures

   C) population

   D) case management

95. A crucial part of case management that contributes to patient autonomy, beneficence, and justice is known as:

   A) veracity.

   B) advocacy.

   C) conduct.

   D) competency.

96. When a CCM exceeds legal duties and adheres to a professional standard, it is referred to as meeting:

   A) acceptable standards.

   B) societal standards.

   C) ethical standards.

   D) appropriate standards.

97. The MOST important aspect of the patient that may affect their health care choices is their:

   A) age.

   B) gender.

   C) spiritual beliefs.

   D) diet.

98. Patients who are ill and practice a spiritual discipline may improve their well-being through all of the following EXCEPT:

   A) improvement of coping skills.

   B) decreasing of suicidal thoughts.

   C) improvement of physical symptoms.

   D) medical education.

99. Assistive devices do NOT include:

   A) tangible items that help disabled persons.

   B) closed captioning and hearing aids.

   C) mobility devices such as a cane or a screen reader.

   D) pacemakers or corneal implants.

100. Your new client is a young man who admits to having depression and some transient suicidal ideation. As you perform your initial case management assessment, you focus on other risk factors for suicide, including:

   A) prior suicide attempts and substance abuse.

   B) socioeconomic status and neighborhood.

   C) family history of depression.

   D) other medical and mental health conditions.

101. Data collected from a number of health care domains and used for analysis is known as:

   A) data analysis.

   B) outcomes measures.

   C) health care analytics.

   D) quality analytics.

102. An example of semantic noise is:

   A) the receiver being too hungry to listen.

   B) terminology the receiver cannot understand.

   C) a startling noise that interrupts the message.

   D) anxiety preventing the receiver from focusing.

103. The following all represent vulnerable populations EXCEPT:

A) the homeless.

B) the uninsured and underinsured.

C) recent immigrants.

D) women.

104. Potential barriers preventing the patient from processing information include all of the following EXCEPT:

A) an educational deficit.

B) cognitive ability.

C) an overload of information.

D) the patient's values.

105. The CCM is also a social worker. When confronted with an ethical dilemma, he knows that he must abide by both his:

A) code of case management and code of conduct.

B) Code of Professional Conduct and code of case management.

C) Code of Professional Conduct and Code of Ethics.

D) code of conduct and code of CCM.

106. Ergonomics improves environmental design by applying all of the following EXCEPT:

A) theory.

B) data.

C) methods.

D) structure.

107. To qualify for home health services, the client must be:

A) financially needy.

B) homebound.

C) non-ambulatory.

D) over age fifty-five.

108. _____ is an insurance that provides wage replacement and medical care to injured employees.

A) Long-term disability

B) Temporary total disability

C) Workers' compensation

D) Workers indemnity fund

109. A process that analyzes data and forecasts probable outcomes is known as:

A) health care analytics.

B) data analysis.

C) outcomes modeling.

D) predictive modeling.

110. A residential treatment facility:

A) is an intermediate care facility for the developmentally disabled.

B) is for end-of-life care for patients with chronic illnesses.

C) is for patients with substance abuse and behavioral illness.

D) is for elderly patients who need assistance with ADLs.

111. URAC is the acronym for:

A) Utilization Review Access Corporation.

B) Utilization Recovery and Credibility.

C) Utilization Review Accreditation Commission.

D) Utilization Review and Care.

112. TRICARE offers a range of health care plans for:

A) disabled veterans.

B) retirees in need of supplemental plans.

C) Medicaid recipients.

D) military personnel.

113. The principles of case management do NOT include:

A) maintaining subjectivity with all patients.

B) placing a patient's interests above the CCM's.

C) obeying regulations.

D) acting with respect and dignity when communicating with other professionals.

114. The item listed below that is NOT typically a component of the health coaching process is:

A) setting goals based on the patient's preferences.

B) building a relationship.

C) motivational interviewing.

D) obtaining MD orders.

115. The Mental Health Parity Act of 1996:

A) excluded substance abuse treatment.

B) had the impact on health insurance plans in practice that it had intended.

C) mandated that mental health benefits be offered in insurance plans.

D) did not mandate that annual insurance plan dollar limits for mental health treatment are equal to medical or surgical benefits.

116. In this sequence, which number is the mode?   4 4 4 4 7 7 10 10 40

A) 4

B) 7

C) 10

D) 90

117. What is NOT true of a person with a chronic illness or disability?

A) They may perform the same work after an illness or disability.

B) They may need a modified work schedule after an illness or injury.

C) They must apply for disability if job modifications cannot be made.

D) They may have their work environment modified after an illness or injury.

118. Your client, a single woman, has had numerous hospitalizations for multiple sclerosis complications and a failed cauda equina surgery and is no longer able to safely ambulate or care for her colostomy. She is stable and ready for discharge. The appropriate level of care would be:

A) an intermediate care facility.

B) an assisted living facility.

C) a skilled nursing facility.

D) palliative care.

119. CMS states that professionals who transition their client to another provider or care setting should:

A) identify the receiving case manager.

B) ensure that the transition is within the same hospital.

C) provide a summary of care record.

D) provide ongoing case management for thirty days.

120. URAC requires case management programs to annually report:

A) five mandatory measures.

B) adverse case outcomes.

C) number of clients served.

D) cost savings.

121. The defining feature of a managed care plan is that it:

   A) employs mechanisms to control utilization of medical services.

   B) allows treatment outside of the network after appeal.

   C) is a less expensive insurance plan.

   D) utilizes more case managers.

122. Important aspects of the introduction phase include all of the following EXCEPT:

   A) informing the patient whom the CCM works for.

   B) explaining the purpose of the interview.

   C) collaborating on patient goals.

   D) inquiring about how the patient wishes to be addressed.

123. All of the following are reasons for establishing a rapport with the patient EXCEPT:

   A) facilitating effective communication.

   B) increasing the likelihood that the patient will disclose personal information.

   C) ensuring the patient will always do what the CCM wishes to improve their health.

   D) increasing patient engagement.

124. The acronym HCFA stands for:

   A) Health Care for All.

   B) Health Care Financing Administration.

   C) Health Continuity for Americans.

   D) Health Care Financial Administrator.

125. The Women's Health and Cancer Rights Act of 1998 did NOT:

   A) require that reconstruction of the unaffected breast is covered to provide symmetry.

   B) require that lymphedema is covered.

   C) state that breast prosthesis is covered.

   D) require reconstruction to be covered for the breast that was removed.

126. The Family and Medical Leave Act (FMLA) does all of the following EXCEPT:

   A) help workers who are expected to be out of work for an extended time.

   B) provide income for workers when they are out of work for an extended time.

   C) allow workers to keep their job after an illness or injury.

   D) allow employees to keep their health insurance while using FMLA.

127. A workers' compensation insurance company employs four case managers. Two spend most of their time in the office, calling employers, injured employees, and providers. The other two accompany injured workers to doctor and therapy appointments. This is best described as:

   A) telephonic and field case management.

   B) office-based and provider-based case management.

   C) disability case management.

   D) workers' compensation case management model.

128. The PAM is:

A) a patient satisfaction survey.

B) a survey to evaluate a patient's ability to manage his own health.

C) a survey used to measure how case management is advocated for the patient.

D) a measure of patient activity after hospitalization.

129. The Pregnancy Discrimination Act states that:

A) an employee on leave with pregnancy-related conditions is not treated the same as a temporarily disabled employee.

B) expenses for pregnancy-related conditions are not covered on the same basis as other health-related conditions.

C) the pregnant employee might have her pay rate decreased while pregnant.

D) the pregnant employee may keep her same job with same pay and insurance when returning to work.

130. A chronic pain treatment program employs a psychologist, rehabilitation counselor, physical therapist, and case manager. They meet every week to discuss their individual findings and goals and to update the team on the status of the client. This is known as a(n):

A) interdisciplinary team.

B) multidisciplinary team.

C) integrated team.

D) clinical treatment team.

131. Your client today at a primary care office has a concussion and a wrist fracture from an assault and robbery outside his condominium complex. He is now home and receiving outpatient neurology and orthopedic care. When you perform your assessment, he tells you he is having trouble sleeping and keeps having "flashbacks" of the incident. You recommend referral to:

A) the sleep clinic at a local hospital.

B) a psychiatrist.

C) a psychologist.

D) no one; you await the doctor's decision.

132. The PAM is:

A) preadmission and management.

B) patient action measures.

C) patient activation measure.

D) patient advocacy model.

133. Health and human services organizations, such as one-stop career centers and aging services centers, can obtain accreditation through:

A) CARF.

B) TJC.

C) URAC.

D) CMS.

134. The term *disability* does NOT refer to:

A) an individual's neurological or physical deviation.

B) a condition that may cause the individual physical or mental challenges.

C) being unable to conduct an activity without certain accommodations.

D) carrying out activities in what is considered a standard way to perform them.

135. Joe, a seventy-nine-year-old veteran, fell at home and sustained a calcaneus fracture. He also has diabetes, is obese, and has had bilateral total knee arthroplasties. These secondary conditions are known as:

A) significant health problems.

B) the medical problem list.

C) the medical history.

D) comorbid conditions.

136. The nonprofit, membership-based organization that works to catalyze improvements in health care with a focus on measures and standards is the:

A) URAC.

B) CARF.

C) NQF.

D) TJC.

137. A developmental disability is NOT:

A) a mental disability that emerged before the age of twenty-two.

B) a physical disability with an onset after the age of twenty-two.

C) a disability that continues indefinitely and limits major activities in life.

D) a traumatic brain injury.

138. A successful health coach realizes that:

A) she needs to convince her patient to do what she wishes to achieve optimum health care goals.

B) she must listen more than she talks.

C) the patient will need to see the primary care physician frequently.

D) the family will be heavily involved.

139. Your client is a forty-eight-year-old injured worker who installs drywall. He is now twenty weeks post rotator cuff and biceps repair and is stalled out in physical therapy, lifting just thirty-five pounds. His job requires him to lift one hundred pounds. You contact the orthopedic surgeon and request consideration for a referral to:

A) a psychologist for counseling.

B) a neurologist for an EMG.

C) another orthopedic surgeon for a second opinion.

D) a work conditioning facility for work-simulated therapy.

140. The quality improvement (QI) cycle begins with:

A) data collection.

B) defining the problem.

C) a sentinel event.

D) a patient complaint.

141. Which statement is NOT true of the Americans with Disabilities Act (ADA)?

A) Cases are determined individually to consider eligibility.

B) The disabled individual is not defined by ADA as being perceived by employers to have a substantially limiting impairment.

C) The disabled employee can be promoted in their job equally to an employee who is not disabled.

D) The disabled employee must be able to meet the employer's job requirements.

142. A special needs trust:

    A) protects assets for disabled individuals without interfering with SSI and Medicaid benefits.

    B) pays for a disabled individual's medical care and negates the need for Medicaid.

    C) protects assets from other family members.

    D) is for anyone who has medical problems and needs to receive SSI and Medicaid benefits.

143. A benefit of a twelve-step program like Alcoholics Anonymous (AA) or Narcotics Anonymous (NA), in addition to long-term effectiveness, is:

    A) it allows participants to chart their own course.

    B) it is a well-known program.

    C) there is no cost to the participant.

    D) it is physician monitored.

144. A highly disciplined, data-intensive methodology for eliminating defects is:

    A) root cause analysis.

    B) black belt.

    C) Six Sigma.

    D) project management.

145. CMS recently promulgated conditions of participation for community mental health centers. These conditions include:

    A) establishing a QAPI program.

    B) providing free services to needy patients.

    C) implementing a CQI program.

    D) offering multiple locations in a state.

146. The process in which a party of a civil lawsuit can obtain relevant information pertaining to his or her case is referred to as:

    A) respondeat superior.

    B) respondeat inferior.

    C) discovery.

    D) subpoena.

147. Medicare Part A provides coverage for:

    A) physical therapy.

    B) hospitalization.

    C) prescriptions.

    D) preventative care.

148. One of the most critical aspects of negotiation is:

    A) being friendly to the other party.

    B) adhering to company guidelines.

    C) being polite but firm in negotiations.

    D) listening actively.

149. To establish the mean, you:

    A) determine the most common number.

    B) average the numbers.

    C) add all the numbers.

    D) establish a range.

150. Knowing the family dynamics of the patient will assist the CCM in all ways EXCEPT:

    A) making referrals for family counseling.

    B) encouraging normal daily routines.

    C) providing interventions for the care plan.

    D) explaining the patient's insurance plan benefits.

ANSWER KEY

1. **B)** Disability case managers manage occupational diseases to return disabled employees to productive employment.

2. **D)** AHRQ is charged with this mission. It is an agency within HHS.

3. **C)** Men and women of average risk are recommended for colorectal screening beginning at fifty.

4. **C)** Although good documentation may serve to guide the family in decision making, the client may not want family or friends to know their activities due to privacy matters.

5. **A)** The Functional Independence Measure (FIM) assesses levels of disability. This tool is composed of eighteen items and seven scales. A 7 on the scale indicates total independence, and 1 is total assistance with care needs.

6. **C)** Part D is the Medicare Prescription Drug Plan.

7. **B)** While many practitioners of Hinduism use Ayurveda—traditional Indian beliefs and methods of medicine—Hinduism does not necessarily prohibit the application of Western medicine.

8. **C)** SSI is for low-income people who qualify by disability, even if they have never worked.

9. **D)** Disease management is not part of family dynamics.

10. **C)** Medications are an important factor when determining a health history, not a patient's role in their family.

11. **B)** An individual must have no more than $2,000 in assets to qualify for SSI, which is needs-based.

12. **C)** The National Healthcare Quality and Disparities Report is the best source for this information.

13. **D)** The measles, mumps, and rubella (MMR) vaccine is not recommended for people born before 1957.

14. **B)** Thirty minutes of moderate physical activity three times per week is a recommended wellness strategy.

15. **C)** The format is not one of the four components of communication.

16. **A)** The patient's spiritual beliefs are the only beliefs with any bearing on their health care needs or the interaction between the CCM and the patient.

17. **B)** This statement sounds biased and may be the opinion of the recorder. Quotation marks are appropriate when documenting facts.

18. **D)** Sleeping is measured by a sleep study, not the Functional Independence Measure (FIM).

19. **D)** SSDI is funded by payroll taxes.

20. **D)** The average days of disability per diagnosis would compare "apples to apples," rather than "apples to oranges" (i.e., comparing days out of work due to carpal tunnel surgery to days out due to total knee arthroplasty).

21. **C)** Women should have a mammogram every year between forty-five and fifty-four.

22. **B)** Communication with the insurer must be included when the CCM is completing documentation.

23. **C)** Although the patient may need to make some changes in order to be healthier,

this is not a component of interpersonal communication.

24. **C)** Background noise is an example of physical interference in interpersonal communication.

25. **D)** The Inpatient Rehabilitation Facility–Patient Assessment Instrument (IRF–PAI) is not solely for Medicaid patients.

26. **A)** The disability must prevent basic work activities or limit earnings to a very low amount established by the SSA, and the disability must be expected to last for at least one year.

27. **C)** Nondisabled people qualify for Medicare at age sixty-five, as long as they have worked enough quarters under Social Security.

28. **A)** A health assessment screening tool can evaluate risks and outcomes and can be descriptive, predictive, or evaluative.

29. **C)** Annual audiology exams are not typically discussed unless requested by the patient's physician.

30. **D)** Although ensuring the safety of the patient is important, telling the caregiver their actions are justified leads to continuation of inappropriate behavior.

31. **B)** Medicare Part B provides coverage for outpatient services such as doctor's visits, screenings, and occupational and physical therapy.

32. **C)** Family involvement in health care decisions is often very important to patients of East Indian origin who are over sixty-five. The CCM should always ask permission from the patient before discussing protected health information (PHI) with anyone, regardless of cultural traditions.

33. **D)** Physical therapy would be documented by the physical therapist, not the CCM.

34. **B)** Own-occupation disability policies are more lenient and expensive than some other policies. Disability may be claimed as long as duties cannot be performed while doing the most recent job.

35. **C)** SSDI recipients must wait two years to receive Medicare. Generally, they receive Medicaid benefits in the interim.

36. **B)** The Agency for Healthcare Research and Quality has identified that rural inhabitants are generally older, poorer, sicker, and more likely to be overweight or obese.

37. **B)** The patient makes the final decision regarding the recommended treatment plan.

38. **A)** Standards of care are statements that define care in the medical community. The patient will be aware of the outcome expected and of care to be received based on scientific knowledge and clinical expertise.

39. **B)** The case manager must be aware of the risk of transitioning care (i.e., medication errors or failure to follow through on a recommended treatment plan).

40. **D)** CHIP is the Children's Health Insurance Program.

41. **A)** This measure is clearly quantifiable and specific as it focuses on a targeted population (discharged COPD patients).

42. **D)** A capitated rate is calculated "per head," or per patient.

43. **A)** The CCM must educate and support the patient's cultural beliefs.

44. **B)** Standards of practice are statements that describe the acceptable level of provider performance based on clinical research and are typically formulated by practitioner organizations.

45. **B)** With an any-occupation long-term disability policy, the premiums are less expensive because the patient must not be able to perform *any* work tasks to qualify for claims.

46. **B)** As of July 2018, forty-nine states have prescription drug monitoring programs (PDMP).

47. **D)** Off-label medication is medication that is being prescribed for a use not defined in the FDA insert.

48. **C)** Readmissions of recently discharged patients are major cost drivers of health care costs, per the AHQR.

49. **C)** According to the teachings of Jehovah's Witnesses, the Bible prohibits blood transfusions.

50. **B)** Standards of care are strict criteria designed for the management of a clinical condition and are not flexible.

51. **C)** Doing what you say you will do builds trust with the patient.

52. **A)** Guided questions help to redirect the interview or to obtain more specific information.

53. **B)** Home health rehabilitation visits are typically two to three times per week.

54. **C)** Explaining the care plan and providing a summary are effective ways for the CCM to close the interview.

55. **C)** The adaption will be more successful if help is accepted.

56. **D)** The potential savings by avoiding a probable ED visit is a soft savings.

57. **C)** Temporary Assistance for Needy Families, administered by US Health and Human Services, provides funding to help support low-income families.

58. **A)** Many people who practice Judaism follow a kosher diet. The CCM should discuss the patient's dietary needs with him or her and arrange for a kosher diet if necessary.

59. **A)** Practice guidelines are recommendations for screenings, diagnostics, and actions to improve the health of the patient.

60. **B)** Perceptual filters describe prejudices of the listener that have been established through their unique experiences, culture, and values.

61. **A)** The medical home is a partnership between primary care doctors and patients and their families that respects the patient's needs and preferences.

62. **A)** Health insurance-based case management is called payer-based case management.

63. **B)** Followers of Judaism, Jehovah's Witnesses, and Christian Scientists may have dietary restrictions, but it is not a common belief among those groups that the diet heals. Practitioners of Traditional Chinese Medicine are more likely to embrace the idea that certain foods can alleviate or cure illnesses.

64. **A)** The evaluation stage is not a goal of motivational interviewing.

65. **B)** Utilization management reviews services for medical necessity, appropriateness, and adherence to quality standards.

66. **B)** Improving return-to-work times and decreasing days out of work is a critical benchmark in workers' compensation.

67. **B)** TRICARE allows military personnel, both active and retired, to receive care at both military and private facilities.

68. **B)** Practicing Muslims traditionally fast during the month of Ramadan. Patients who are Muslim and have diabetes should speak with their health care provider before Ramadan starts to ensure that they are meeting their medical needs.

69. **B)** Clinical pathways use evidence-based guidelines to incorporate common diseases and procedures into an algorithm format.

70. **D)** Nodding is a customary way to greet someone and is a sign of respect in Chinese culture.

71. **A)** A speech pathologist is trained to evaluate swallowing as well as speech, fluency, and the effects of cognition on speech.

72. **C)** The job schedule is not a factor with the functional job analysis.

73. **C)** On average, people who are spiritual live a longer life.

74. **B)** Support groups can be an important psychosocial resource.

75. **B)** A preferred provider organization (PPO) is a network of providers that agrees to provide services for a lower reimbursement rate and offers users more freedom to select providers.

76. **C)** Studies have demonstrated that, statistically, the chances of return-to-work decrease dramatically as time out of work continues.

77. **B)** The Leapfrog Group is a national nonprofit that conducts outcome surveys and provides a hospital report card for consumers.

78. **C)** Care coordination is the implementation phase of a case management plan, as defined by the Case Management Body of Knowledge (CMBOK).

79. **A)** Evidence-based practice refers to the use of medical interventions proven by research to be effective.

80. **A)** Autonomy describes personal freedom of the patient to make their own choices in health care decisions.

81. **A)** Transitional Work Duty (TWD) allows an injured worker to perform a work task at a lower capacity than prior to injury.

82. **C)** The premium is the monthly cost of insurance.

83. **D)** Case managers are mandatory reporters in most statutes, and elder neglect/abuse must be reported to the appropriate agency in the jurisdiction for further investigation.

84. **C)** The Joint Commission is charged with this responsibility.

85. **B)** The CCM should always use open-ended questions when initiating an interview.

86. **D)** Creating goals for the patient's health needs comes at the end of the interview and is a collaborative process between the CCM and the patient.

87. **D)** This case manager performs disease management. The other answers are contrived definitions.

88. **C)** The term *veracity* describes the act of telling the truth.

89. B) Ergonomics refers to the understanding of human interactions and systems. Ergonomists design and evaluate products that address issues related to environment, productivity, and operator fatigue.

90. C) Language skills, representation, and cultural sensitivity are components of cultural competence, but the definition of *cultural competence* includes multiple factors like race, ethnicity, language, and socioeconomic status.

91. C) This is transition of care, as defined by the Case Management Body of Knowledge (CMBOK).

92. D) Community health centers were created to treat underserved populations.

93. B) Mortality is one of the most important measures evaluated by CMS.

94. A) Process measures are the steps in a process that translate to a negative or positive outcome.

95. B) Patient advocacy is a main factor in case management that fosters patient autonomy, justice, and beneficence.

96. C) Adhering to ethical standards means exceeding legal duties and following an even higher standard.

97. C) Patients' spiritual beliefs could directly impact their choices regarding medical care.

98. D) Spirituality does not impact medical education.

99. D) Assistive devices are external.

100. A) The Substance Abuse and Mental Health Services Administration (SAMHSA) identifies prior suicide attempts and substance abuse as risk factors, along with access to lethal weapons.

101. C) Health care analytics is the term for health care analysis activities derived from data collection from four areas.

102. B) Medical terminology that the receiver cannot understand is an example of semantic noise. The CCM must realize that semantic noise impacts the patient's ability to engage.

103. D) Being a woman does not necessarily equate with being part of a vulnerable population.

104. D) The patient can still process information even if their value system is different from the CCM's.

105. C) He must abide by the CCMC's Code of Professional Conduct as a CCM, and the Code of Ethics as a social worker.

106. D) Principles, along with theory, data, and methods are applied in ergonomics to improve environmental design.

107. B) The client must be homebound or have significant difficulty leaving the home to qualify for home health services.

108. C) Workers' compensation provides these benefits in exchange for the surrender of the ability to sue the employer through the tort system.

109. D) Predictive modeling uses statistics to predict outcomes.

110. C) A residential treatment facility is an inpatient facility for treatment of substance abuse and other mental and behavioral disorders.

111. C) URAC, the Utilization Review Accreditation Commission, accredits a number of professional organizations.

112. D) TRICARE, formerly CHAMPUS, provides a range of health care plans for active and retired military personnel.

113. A) Maintaining *objectivity* with all patients is a principle of case management.

114. D) The goal of the health coach is to achieve patient-related goals. Obtaining MD orders is not part of their role.

115. A) Substance abuse and chemical dependency are not covered under this act.

116. A) Four is the most commonly listed number, so this is the mode.

117. C) If job modifications cannot be made after an injury or illness, the worker may change jobs or apply for disability, but applying for disability is not required.

118. C) This client should go to a skilled nursing facility, which provides twenty-four-hour skilled care and rehabilitation. The other choices would not provide an adequate level of skilled care, given the diagnoses and current level of functioning.

119. C) A summary of care should be provided at each transition/referral to reduce the chances of an adverse outcome.

120. A) URAC requires accredited case management organizations to report on five mandatory measures.

121. A) Managed care plans use various techniques to limit or control patient access to medical services. These techniques may include referrals, contracts with medical providers, and requiring approval for certain medical services.

122. C) Collaborating on goals is important but is not part of the introduction phase.

123. C) Despite a good rapport, the patient may not always do what the CCM wishes to improve their health.

124. B) HCFA is the Health Care Financing Administration, a division within the US Department of Health and Human Services.

125. C) Mastectomy coverage does not include breast prosthesis.

126. B) The Family and Medical Leave Act (FMLA) does not provide income.

127. A) Telephonic and field case management are the appropriate definitions of these functions.

128. B) The patient activation measure evaluates the knowledge, skills, and confidence patients need to manage their own health care.

129. D) No employment discrimination is allowed because an employee is pregnant. This means the employee may keep her same job with same pay and insurance when returning to work.

130. B) This is a multidisciplinary team because people from different disciplines are working together but drawing from their own individual expertise. An interdisciplinary team is similar but involves team members working as an integrated whole, often with overlapping roles and goals.

131. C) A psychologist is best suited to provide cognitive and behavioral therapy. Since the client told you about these symptoms, it is appropriate to make this recommendation to the physician. The psychologist may recommend the patient see a psychiatrist for further treatment with medication, but the case manager should suggest referral to a psychologist first.

132. C) The patient activation measure is a commonly used measure to assess a patient's ability to manage her health care.

133. **A)** The Commission on Accreditation of Rehabilitation Facilities, CARF, is the accrediting body for health and human services organizations.

134. **D)** A disability may be described as the inability to perform activities in what is considered a standard way for a person to carry them out.

135. **D)** Comorbid conditions such as Joe's are usually long-term and chronic.

136. **C)** The National Quality Forum, NQF, has done extensive work in continuous quality improvement and has an endorsement process for health care measures.

137. **B)** A physical or mental disability must emerge before age twenty-two to be considered a developmental disability.

138. **B)** A successful health coach will need to listen to the patient and set goals based on the patient's conversations.

139. **D)** A work conditioning facility will provide more aggressive and individualized therapy that simulates work.

140. **B)** The first step in QI models is defining the problem or area to be studied.

141. **B)** The disabled individual is defined by the Americans with Disabilities Act (ADA) as being perceived by employers to have a substantially limiting impairment.

142. **A)** The trust names a trustee as administrator; since the disabled individual does not have direct access to the funds, it protects the individual's ability to receive SSI and Medicaid.

143. **C)** Alcoholics Anonymous (AA) and Narcotics Anonymous (NA) are free and operate with member donations only, providing a proven outpatient treatment model at no cost.

144. **C)** Six Sigma is a methodology that drives to attain six deviation points between mean and nearest specification.

145. **A)** Community mental health centers must develop and implement a Quality Assurance Performance Improvement Program (QAPI) as established by CMS in its 2014 regulations.

146. **C)** *Discovery* is the term used to describe the process in which a party of a civil lawsuit can obtain relevant information pertaining to his or her case.

147. **B)** Medicare Part A provides coverage for inpatient hospital care, inpatient skilled nursing care, and hospice care.

148. **D)** Active listening involves listening to the other party to find possible areas of compromise.

149. **B)** The mean is obtained by averaging the numbers (i.e., adding all numbers and dividing by the number of numbers).

150. **D)** The CCM may educate the patient or family member about insurance plan benefits without knowing the family dynamics.

Follow the link below for your second CCM practice test:

www.ascenciatestprep.com/ccm-online-resources

CPSIA information can be obtained
at www.ICGtesting.com
Printed in the USA
LVHW061413200720
661129LV00016B/828

9 781635 305449